COLOR THE FUNNY & SNARKY PHARMACY TECH QUOTES WITH MANDALA PATTERNS

Nothing scares me i'm a PHARMACY TECHNICIAN

PHARMACY TECHNICIAN

COLORING BOOK FOR ADULTS

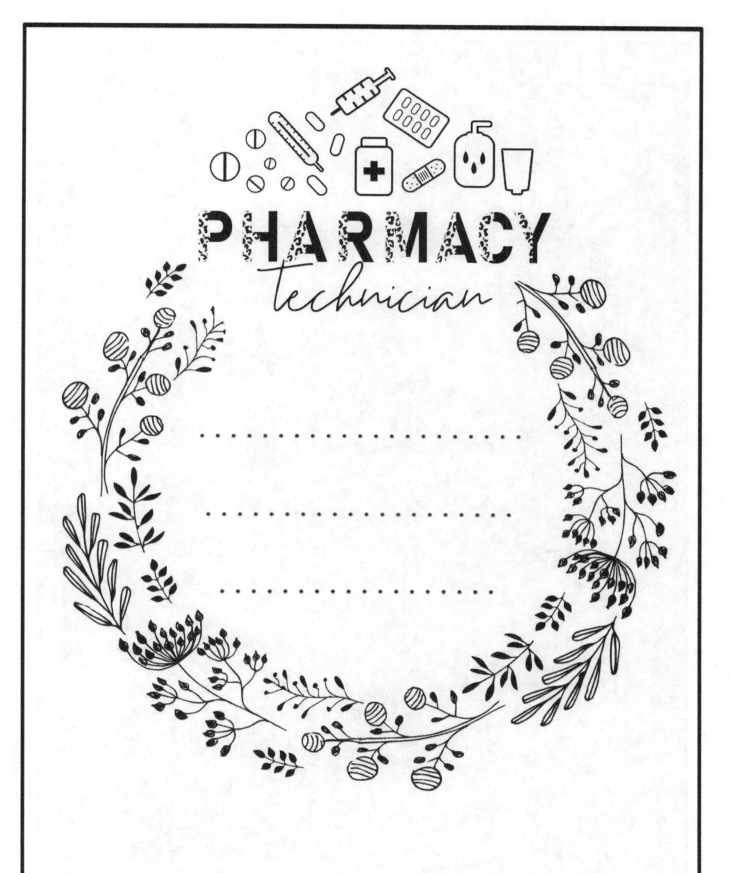

PHARMACY
technician

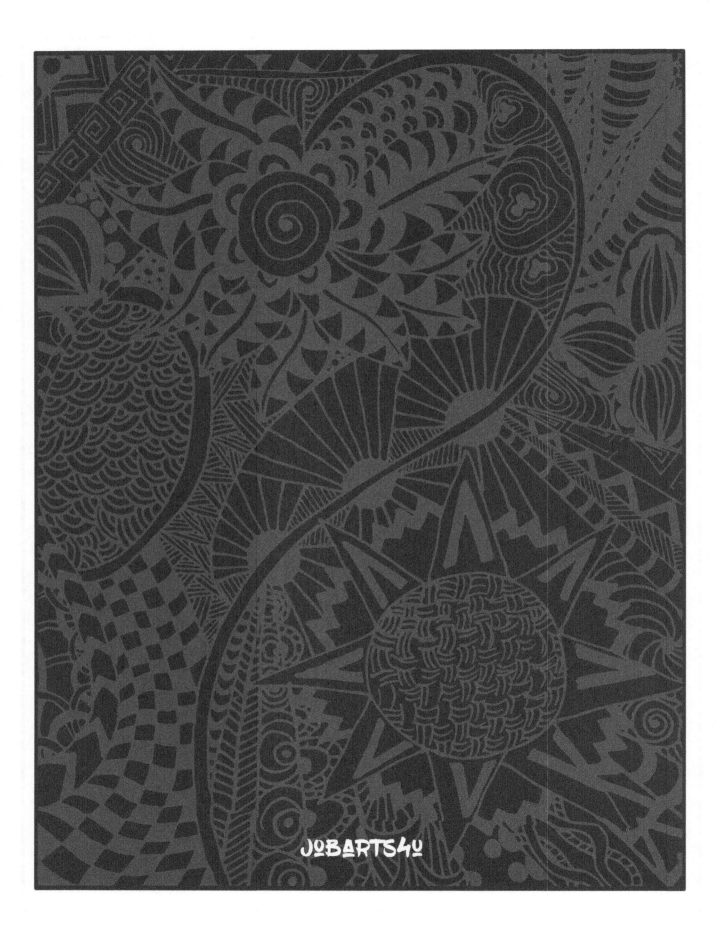

TEST THE COLORS HERE

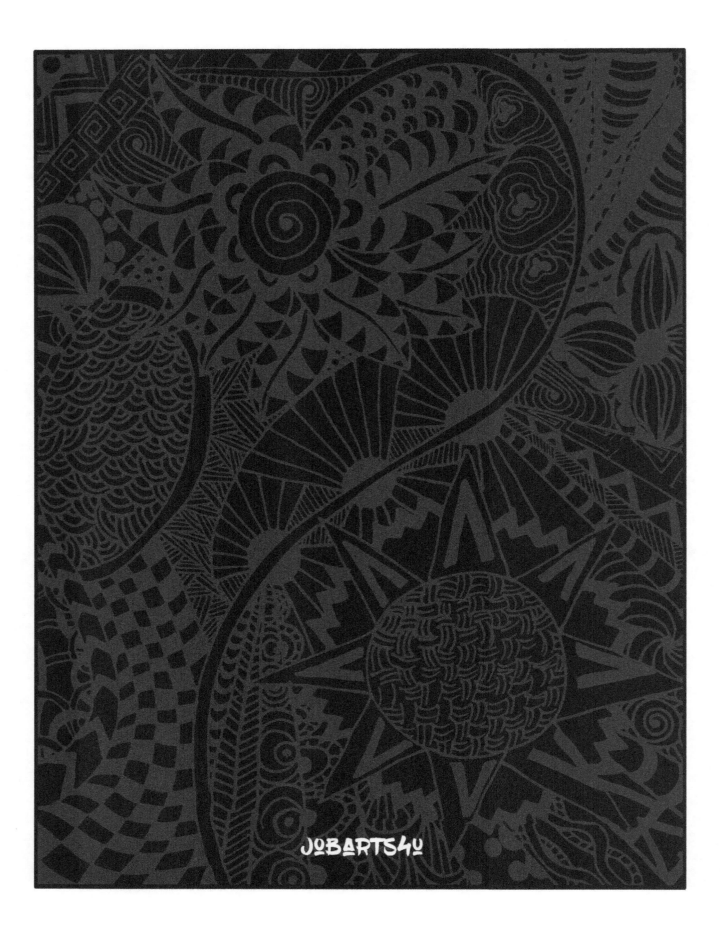

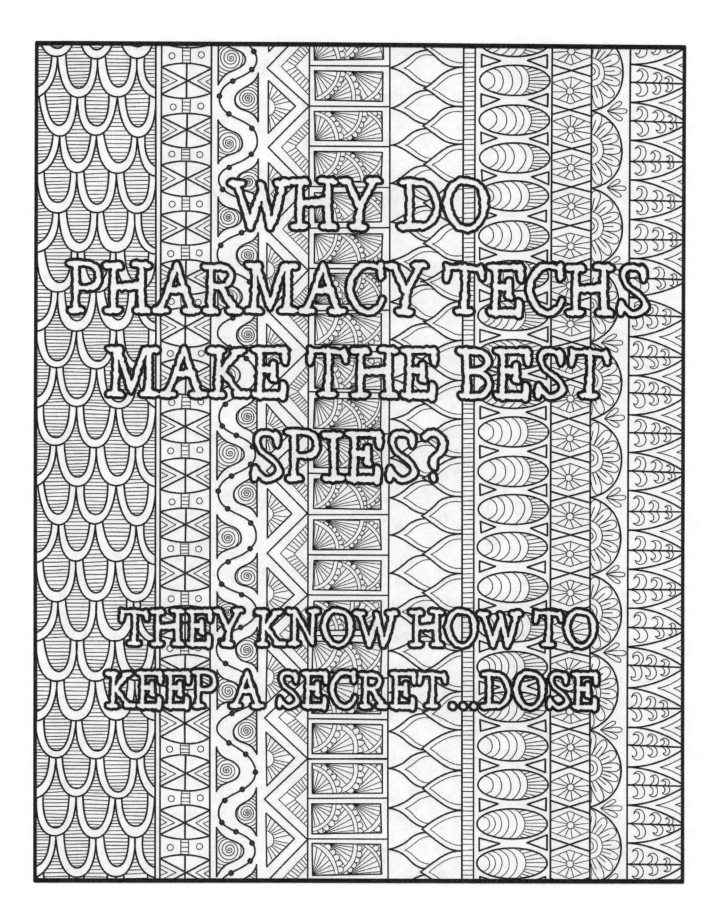

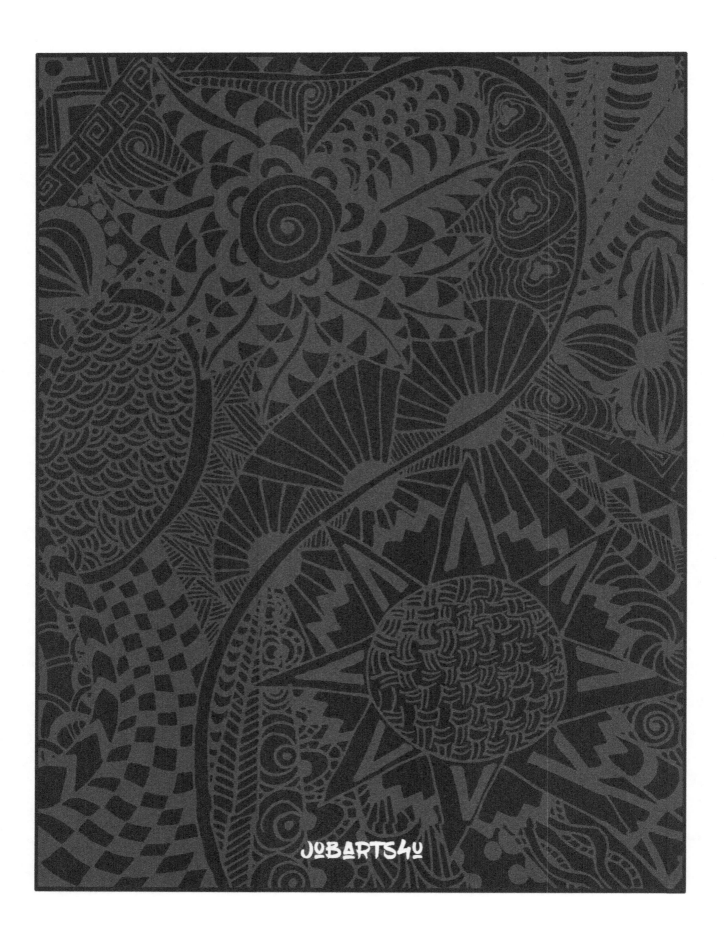

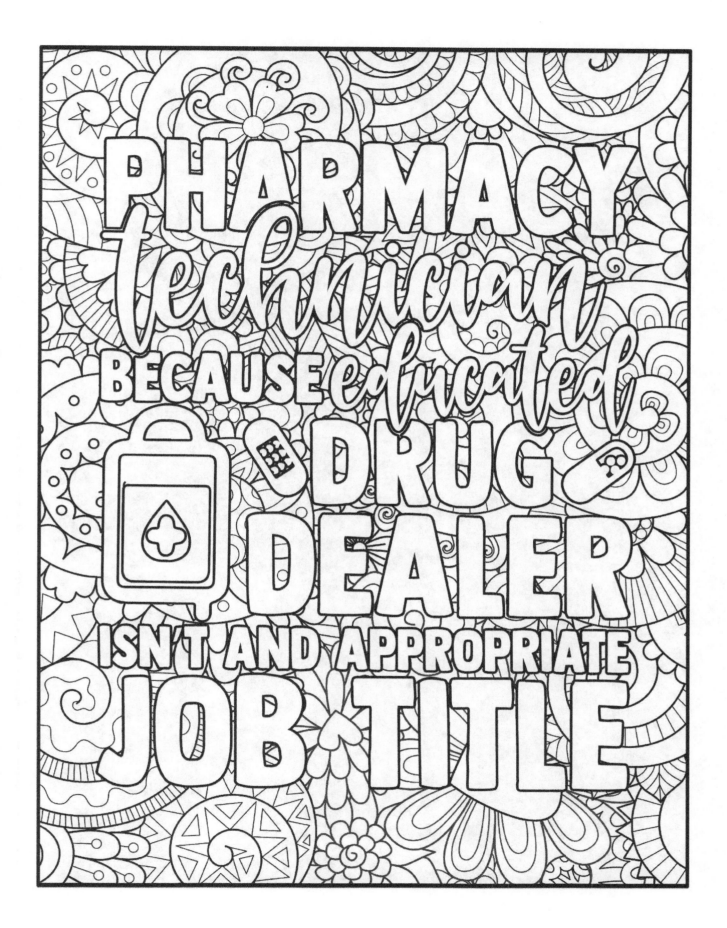

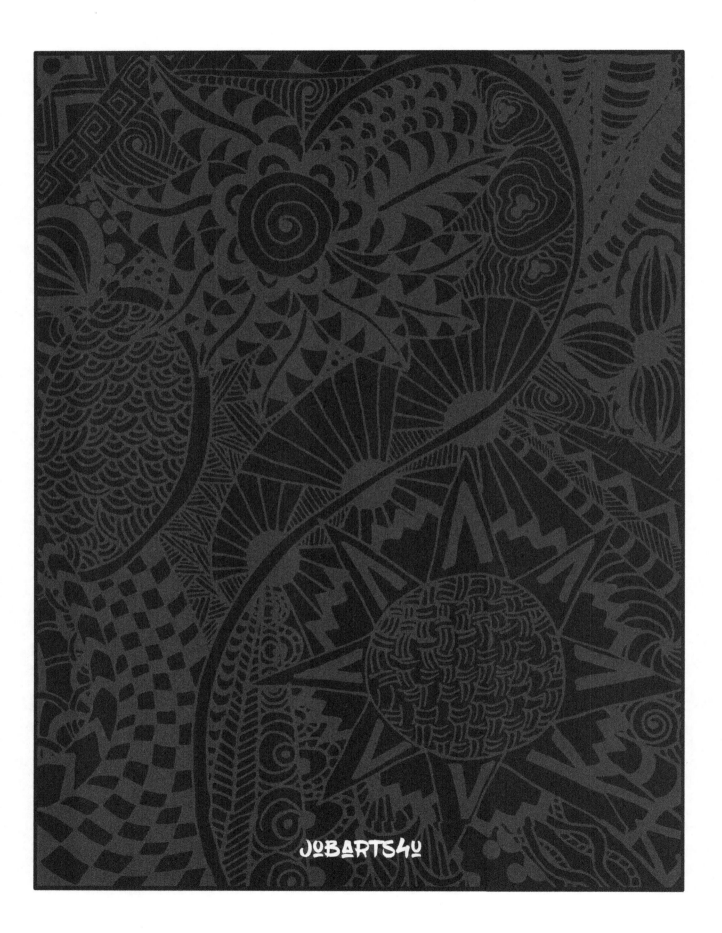

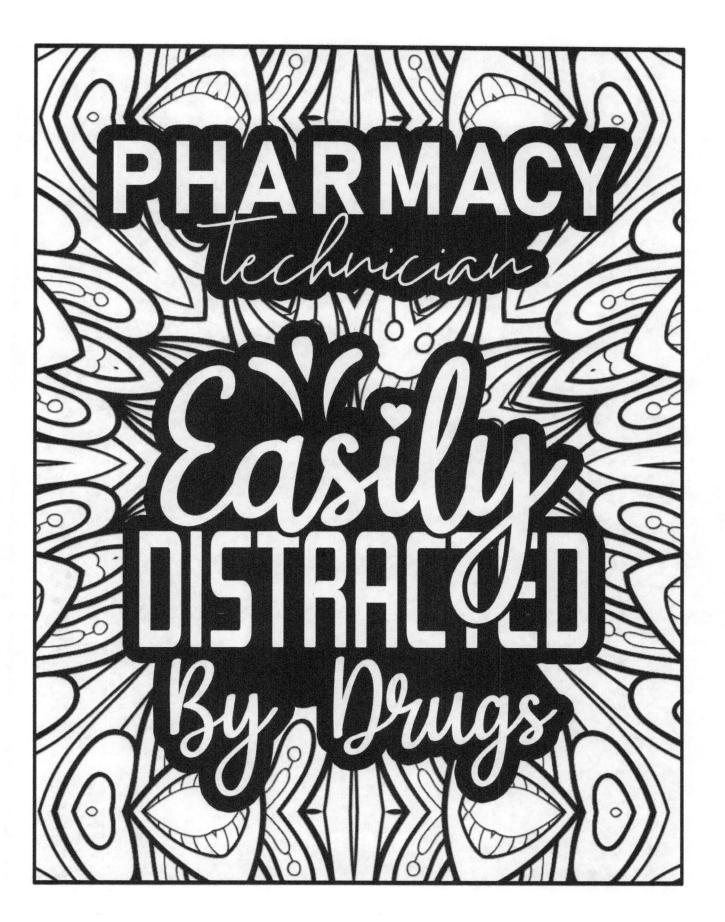

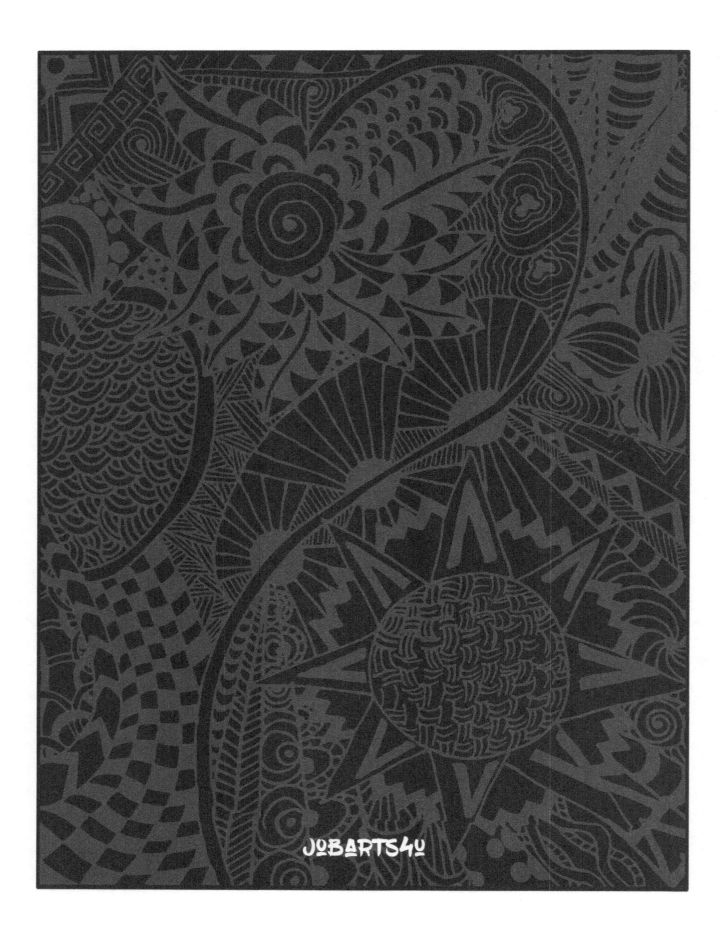

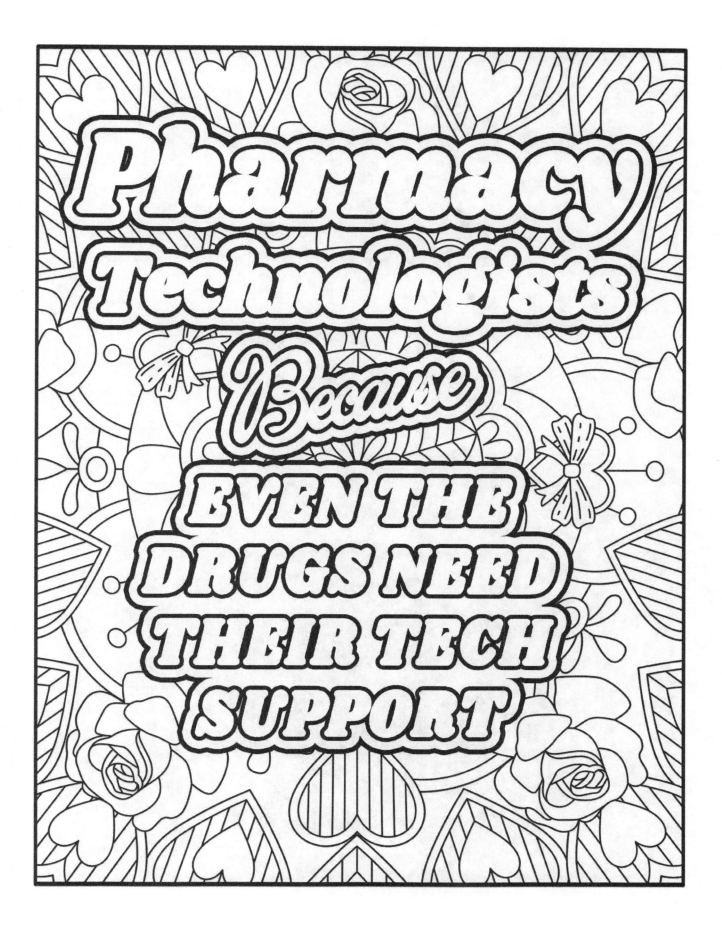

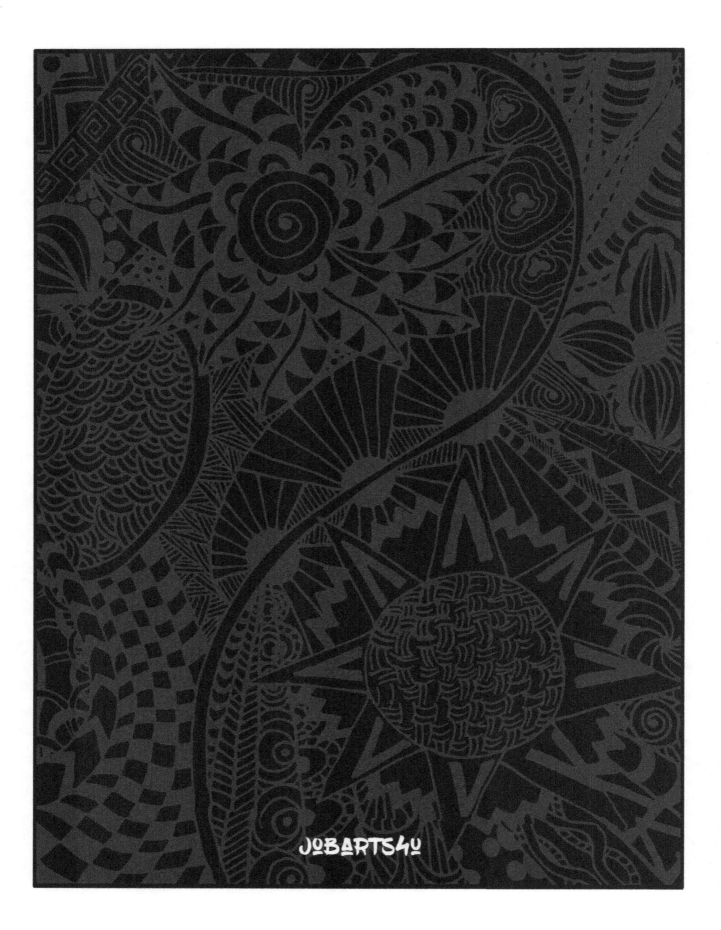

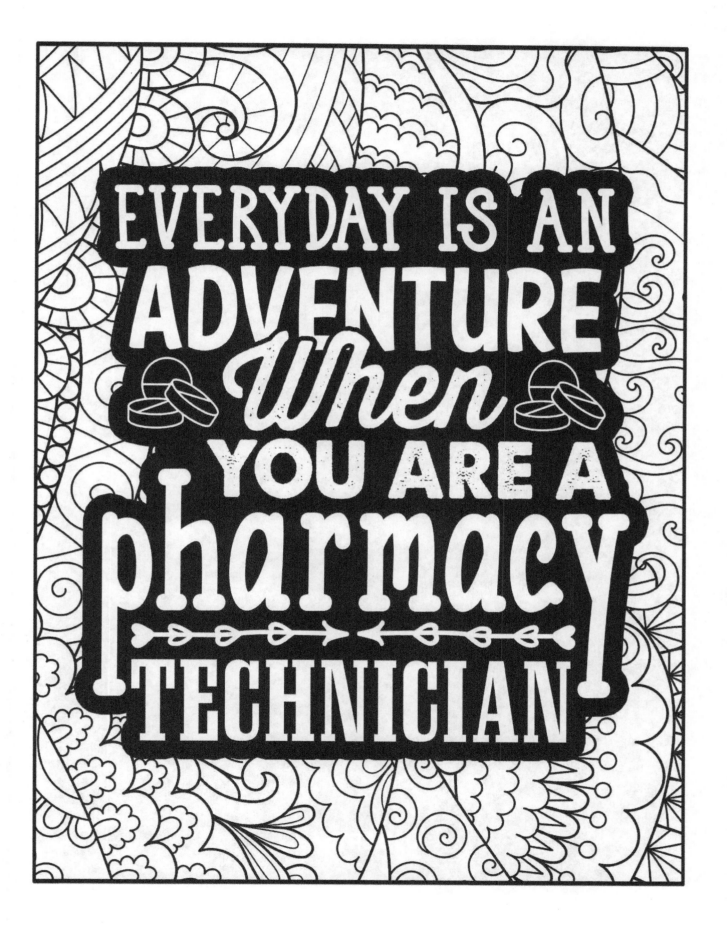

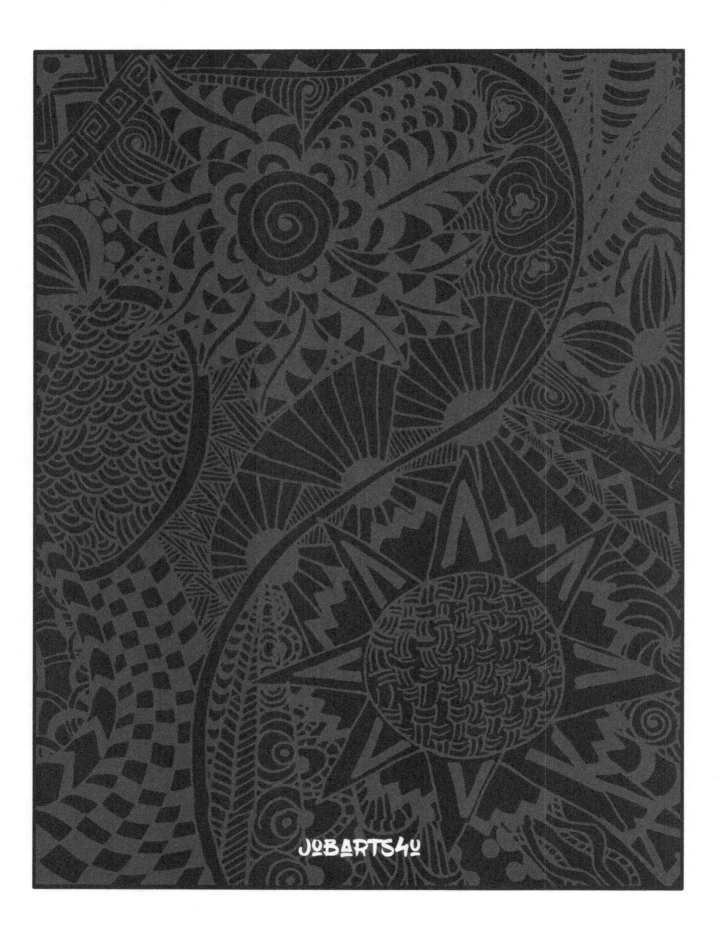

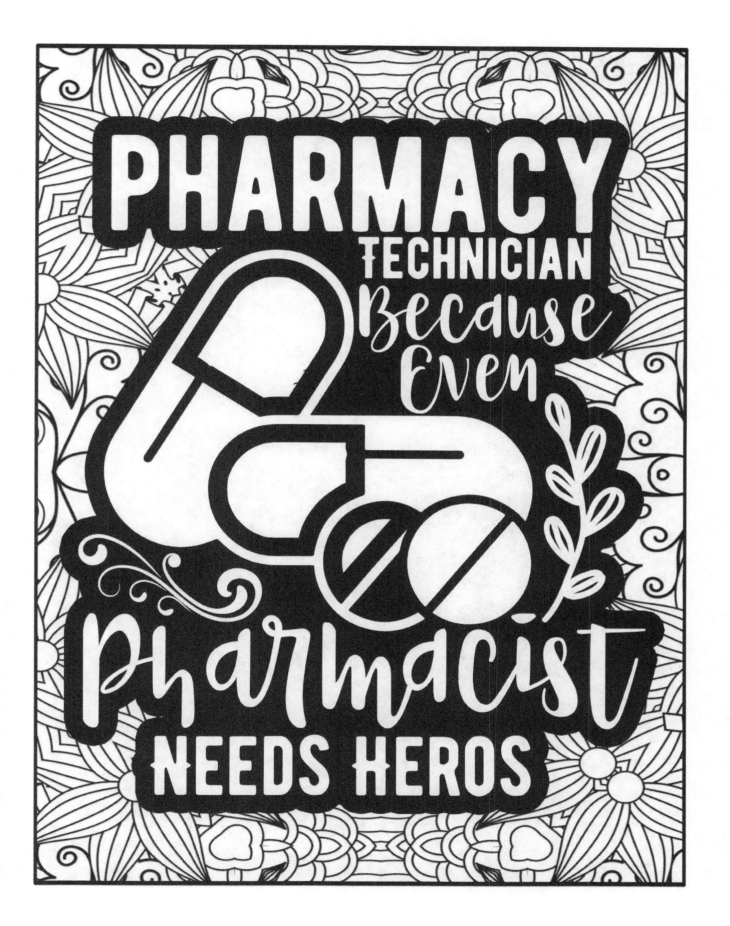

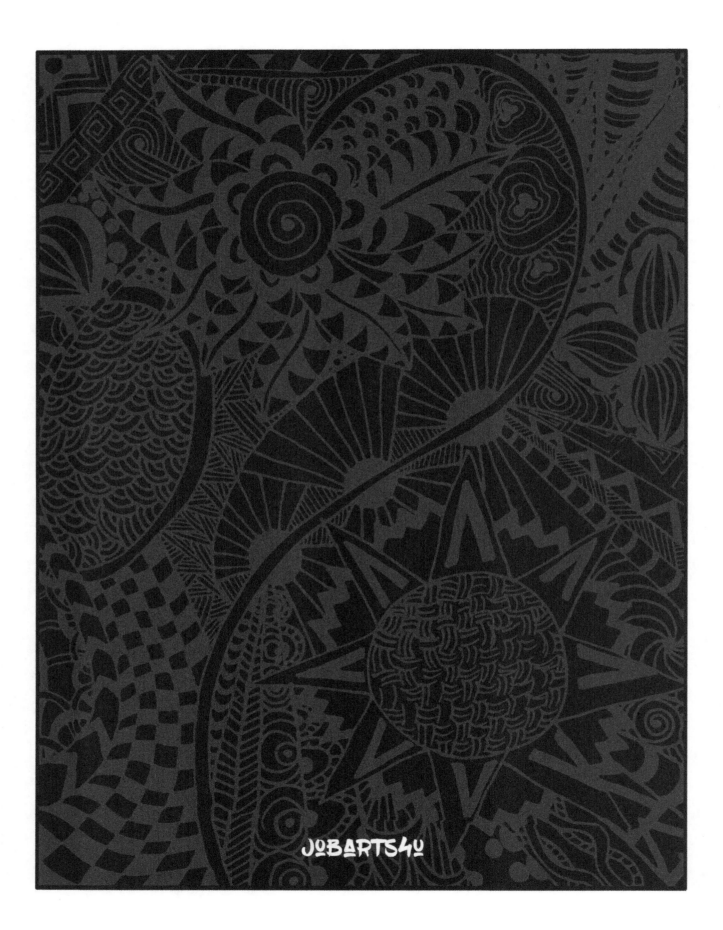

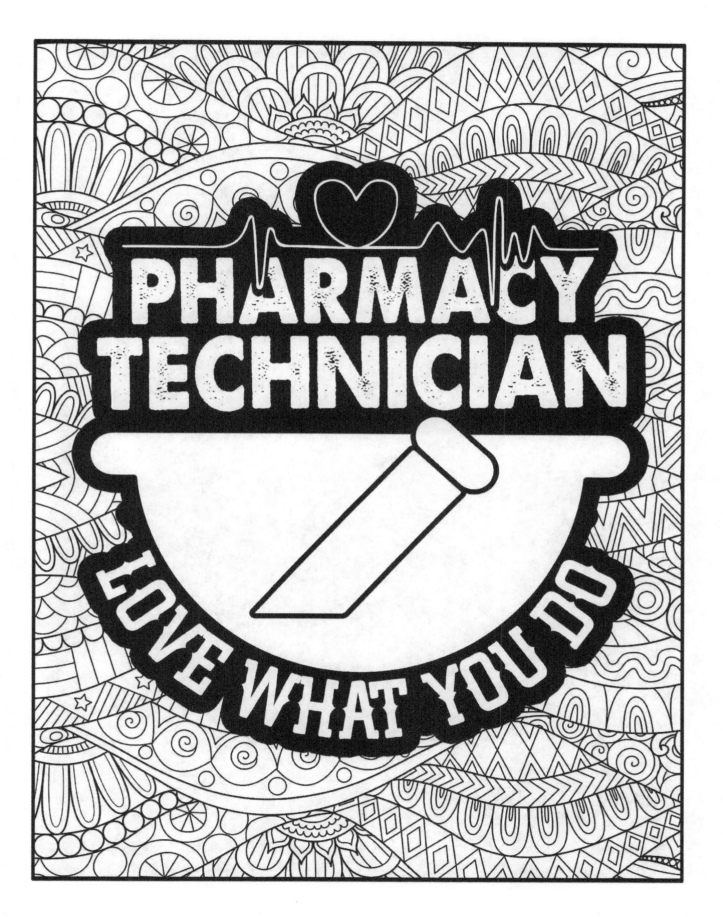

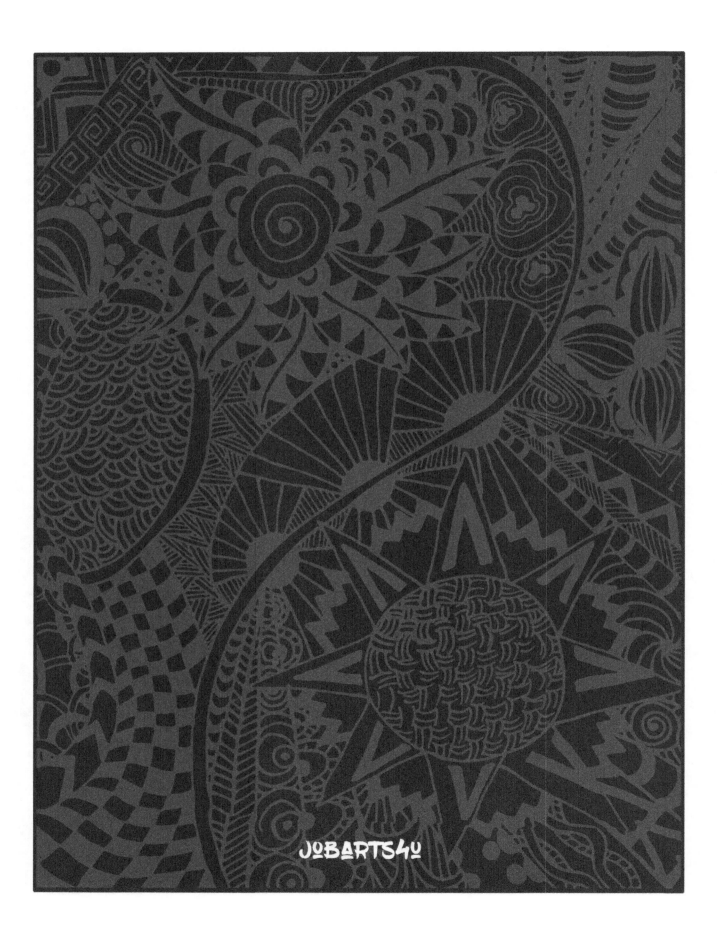

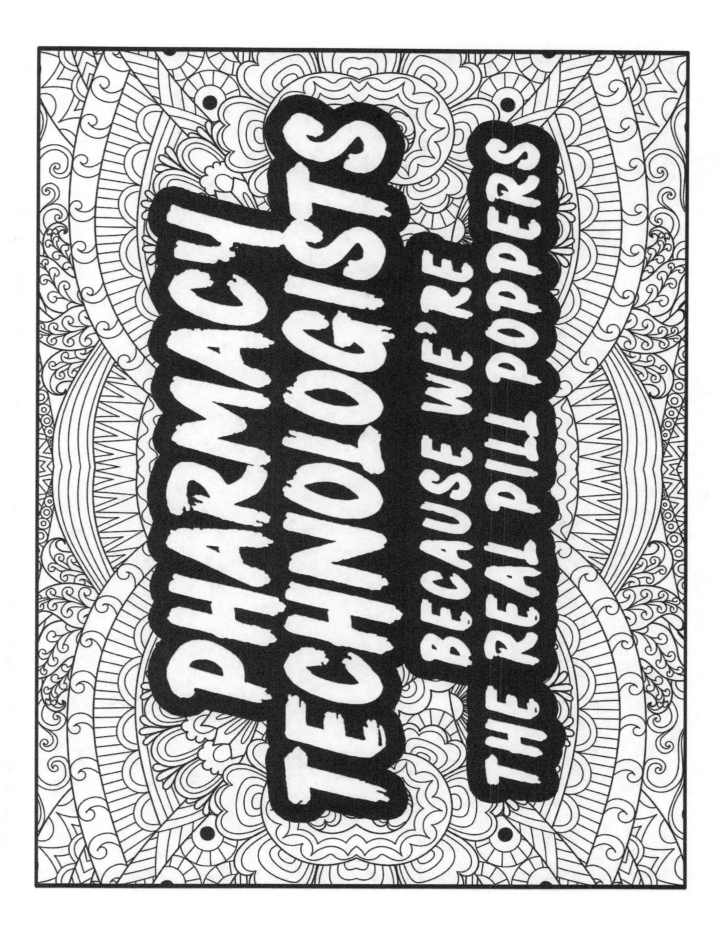

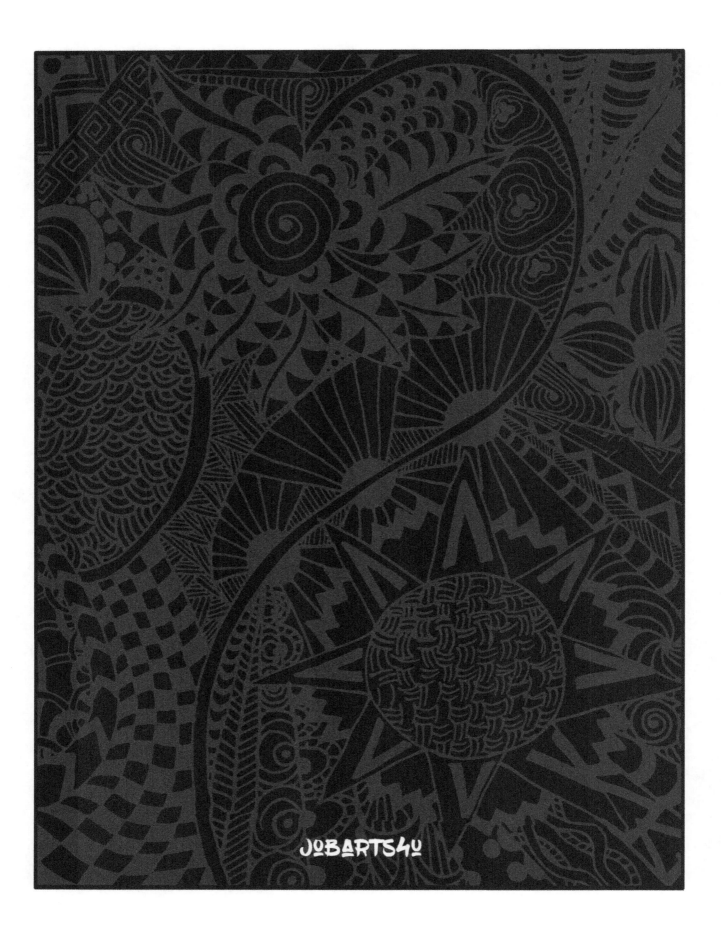

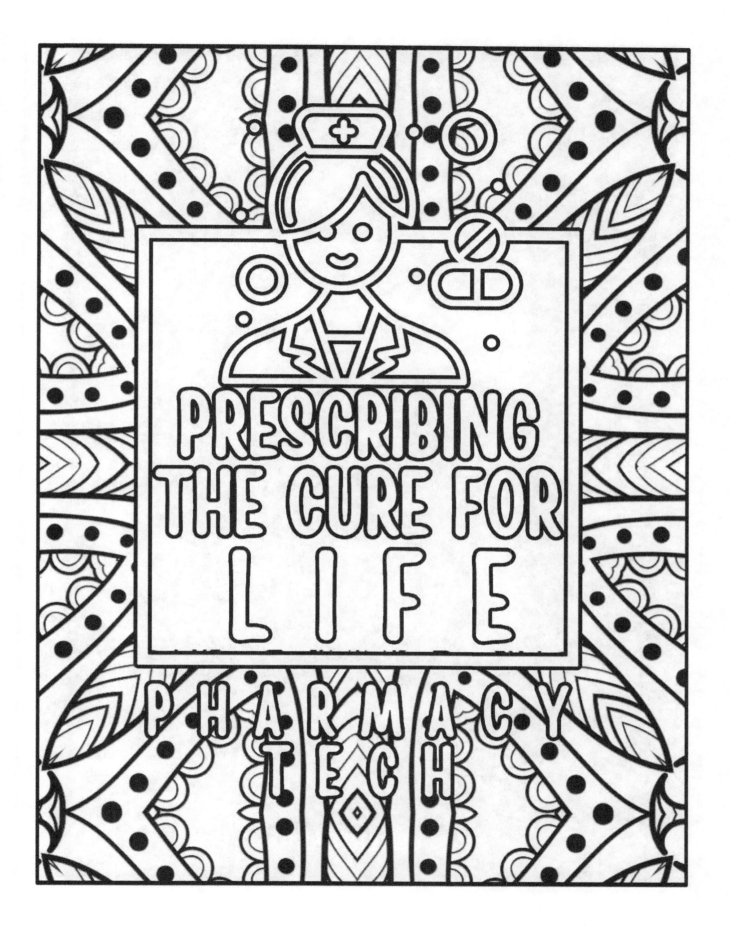

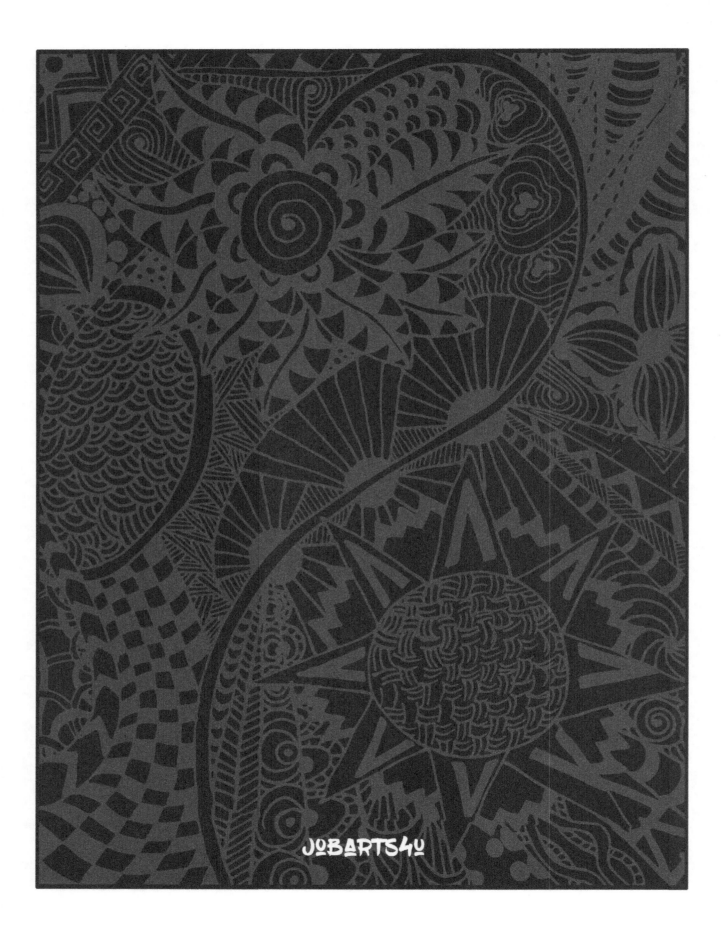

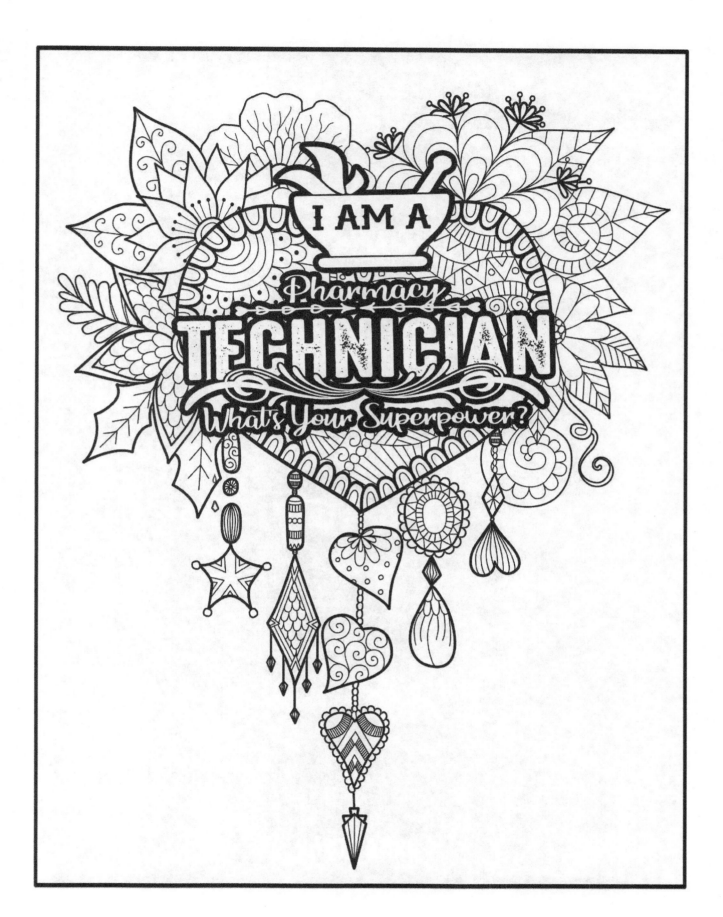

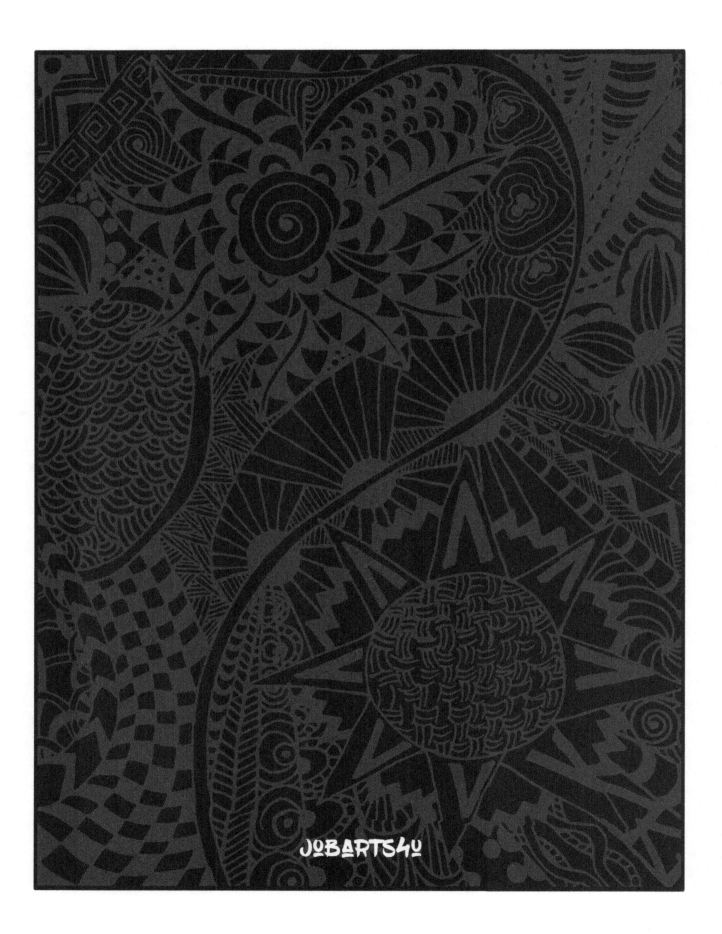

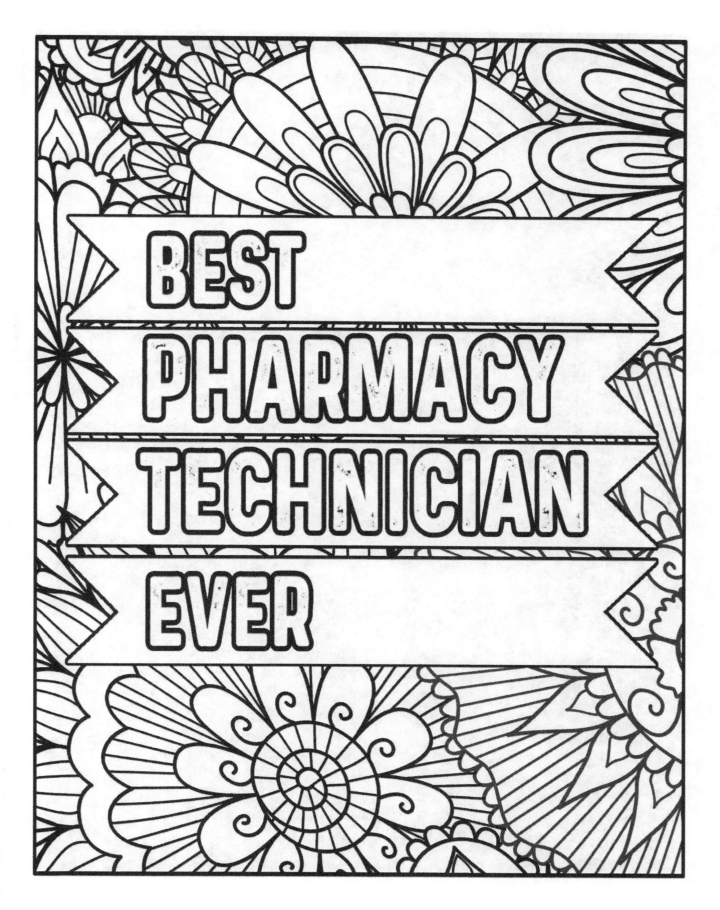

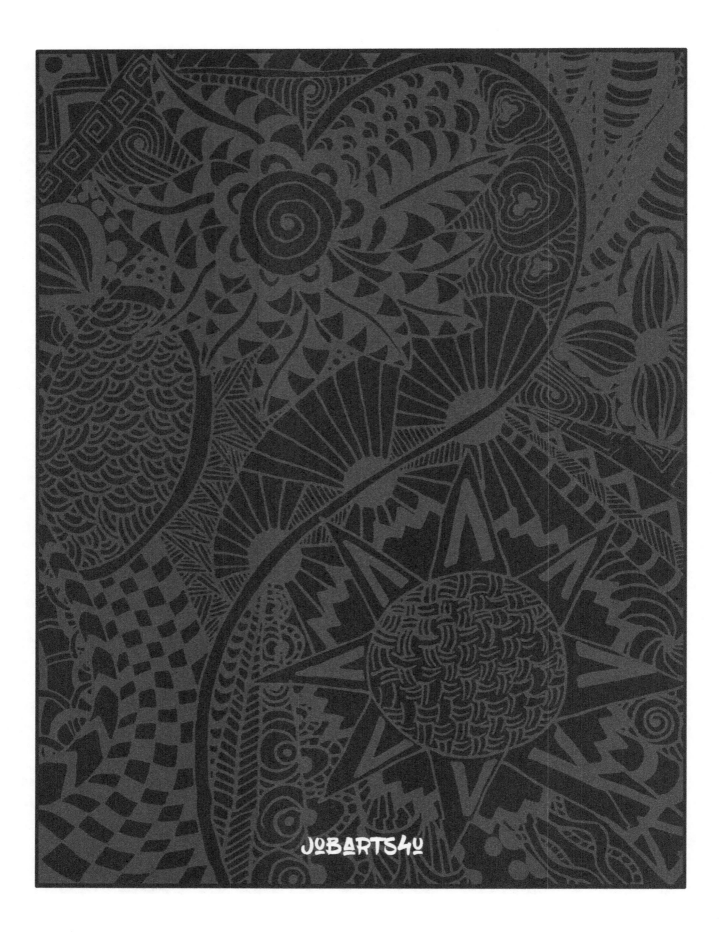

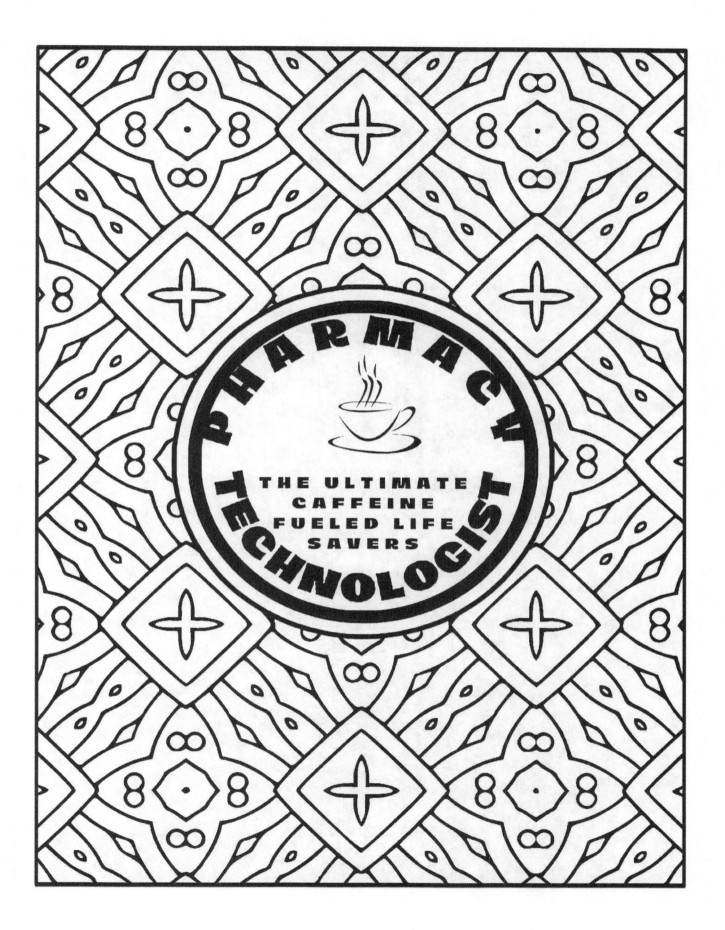

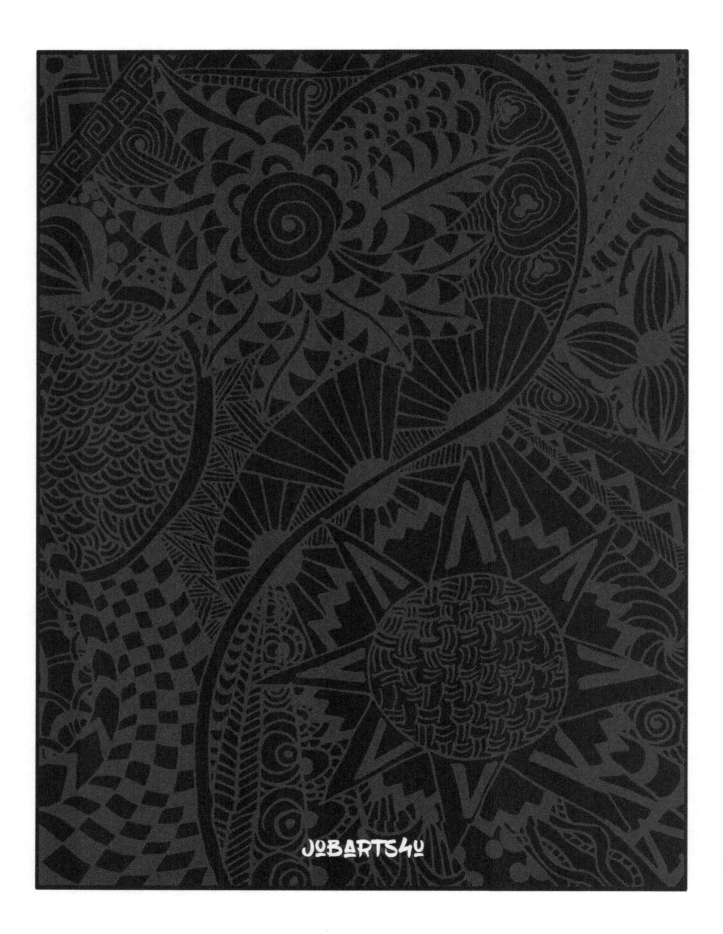

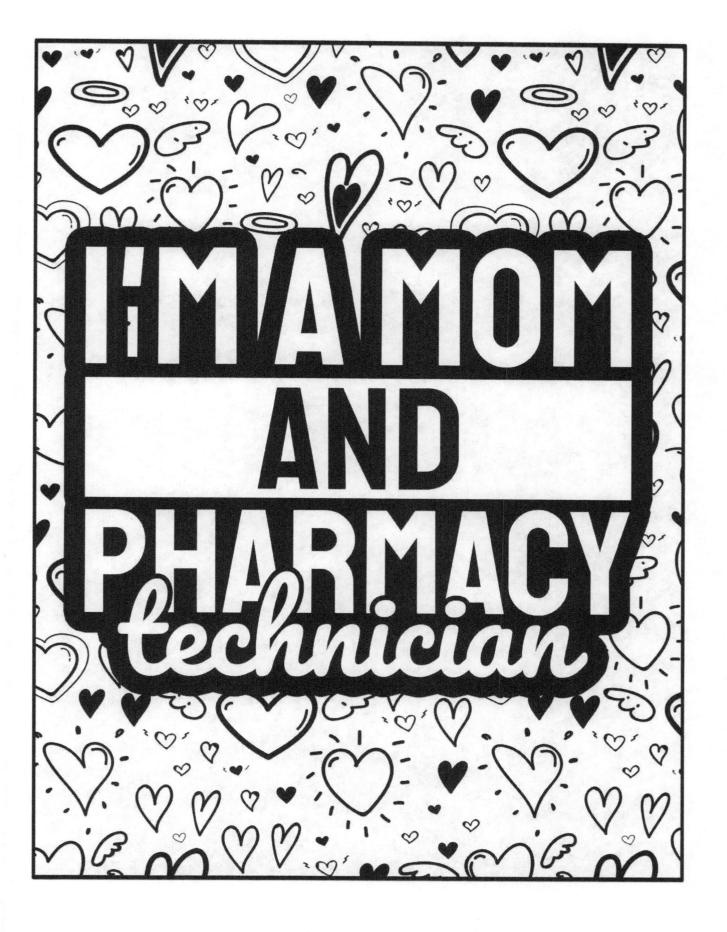

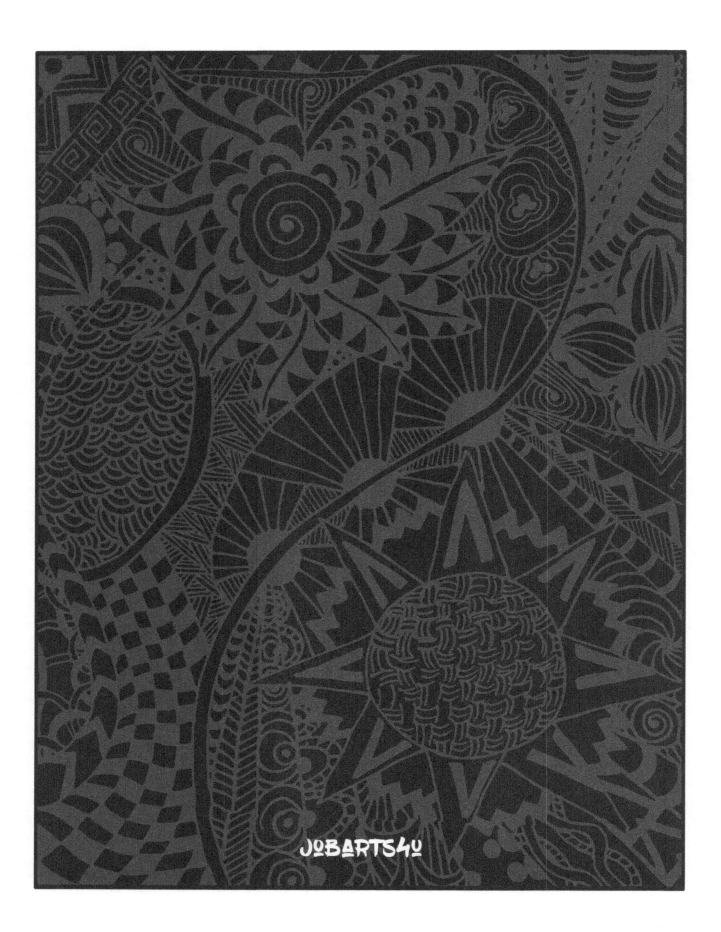

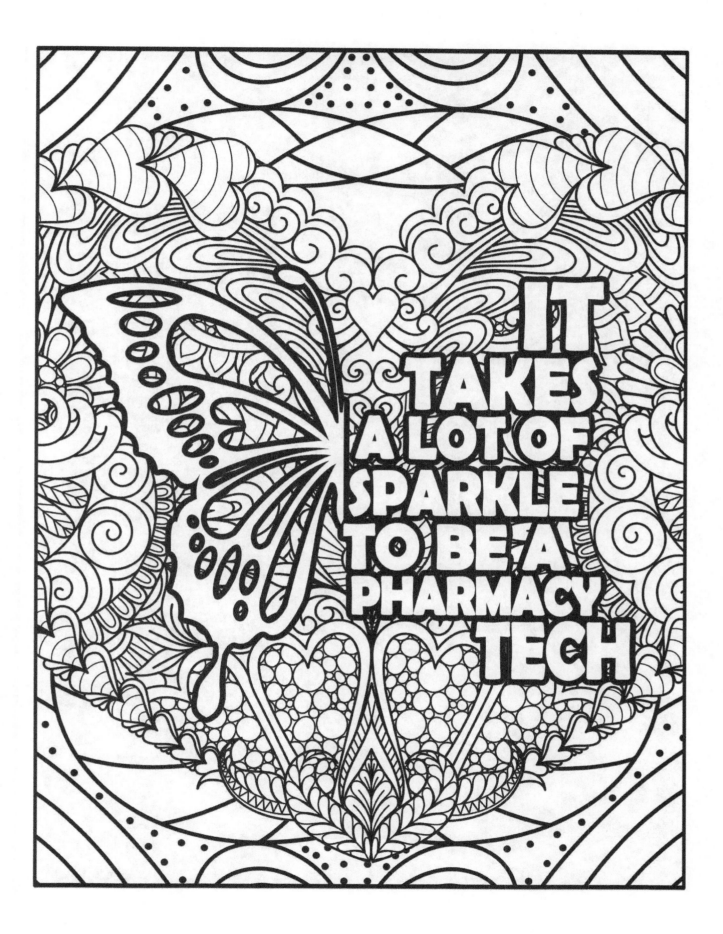

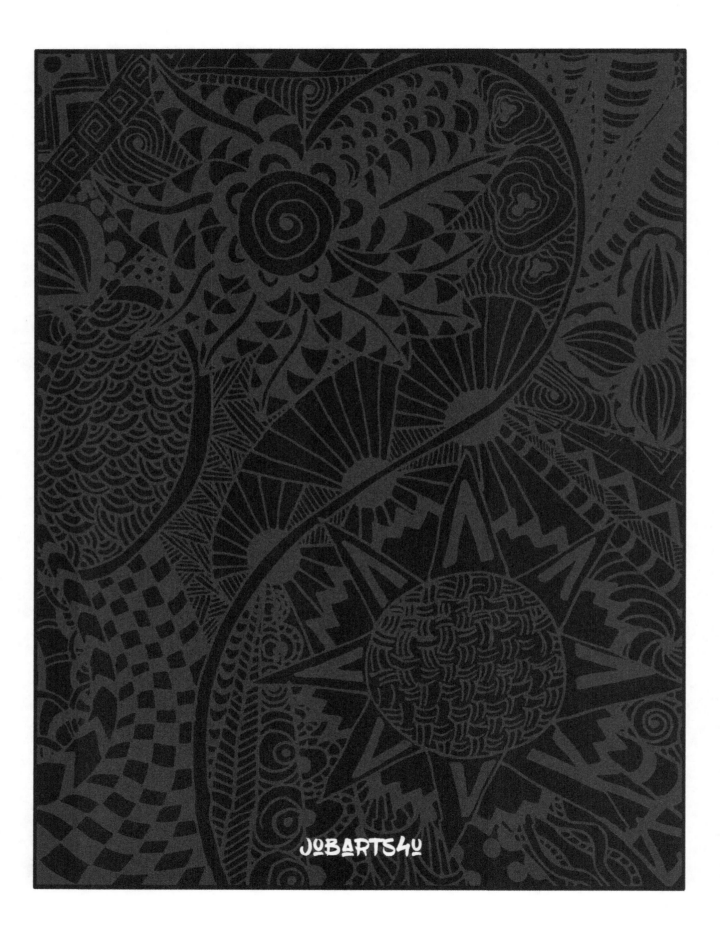

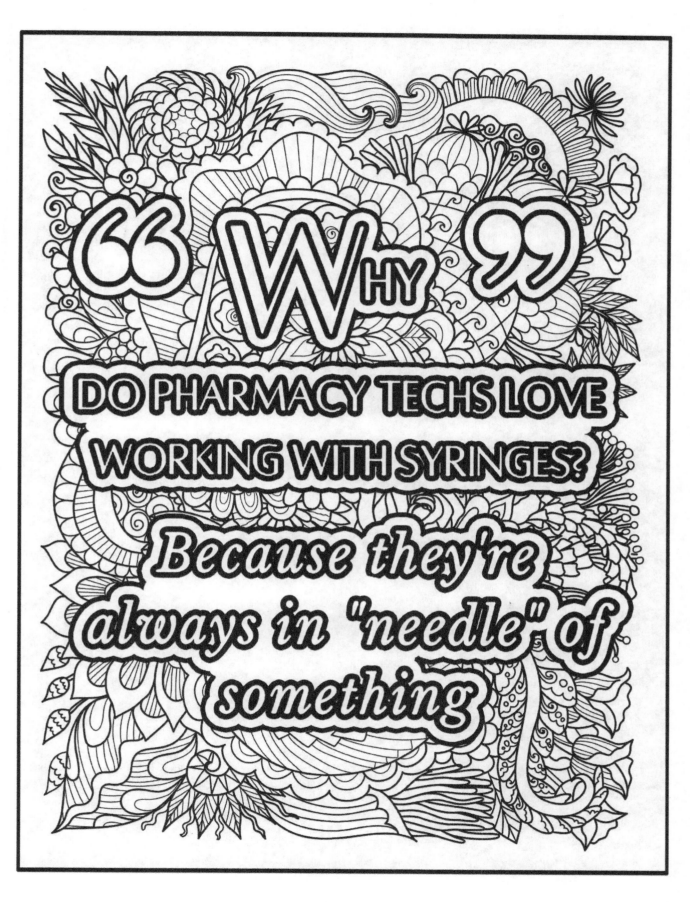

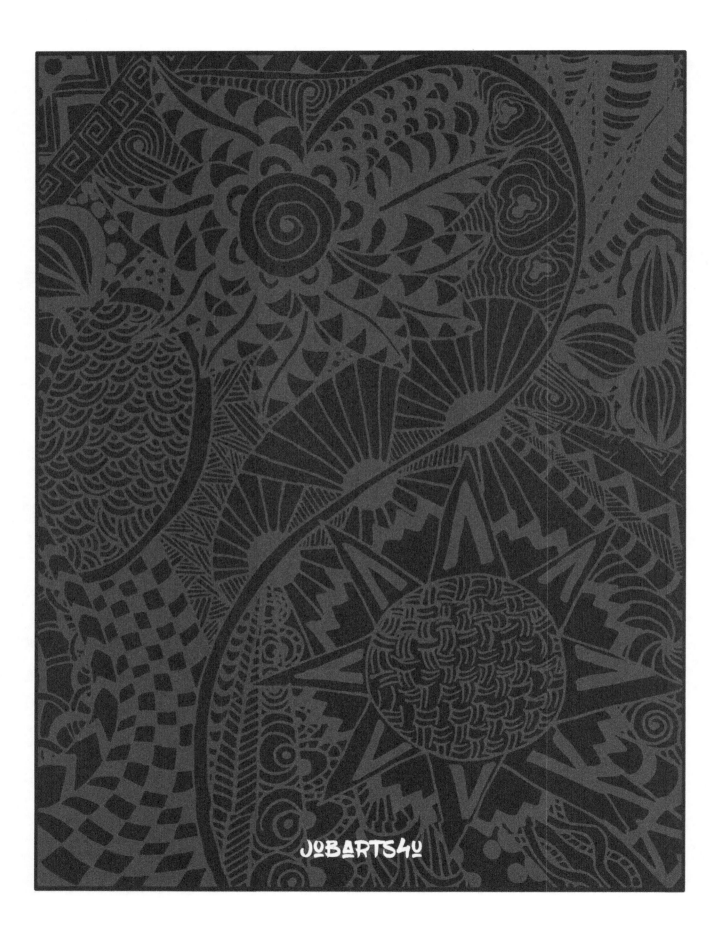

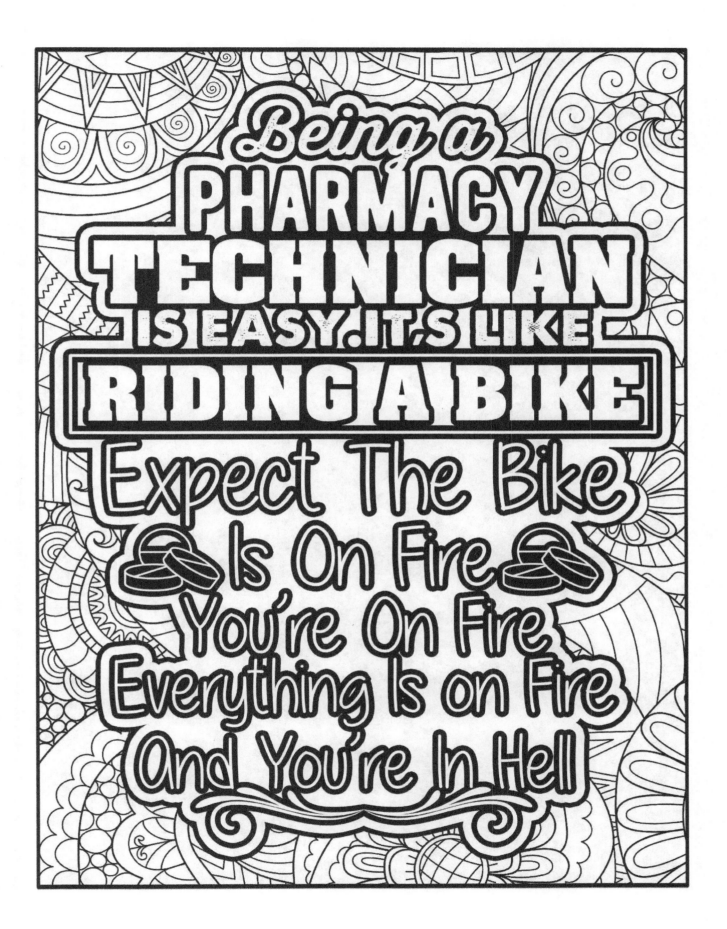

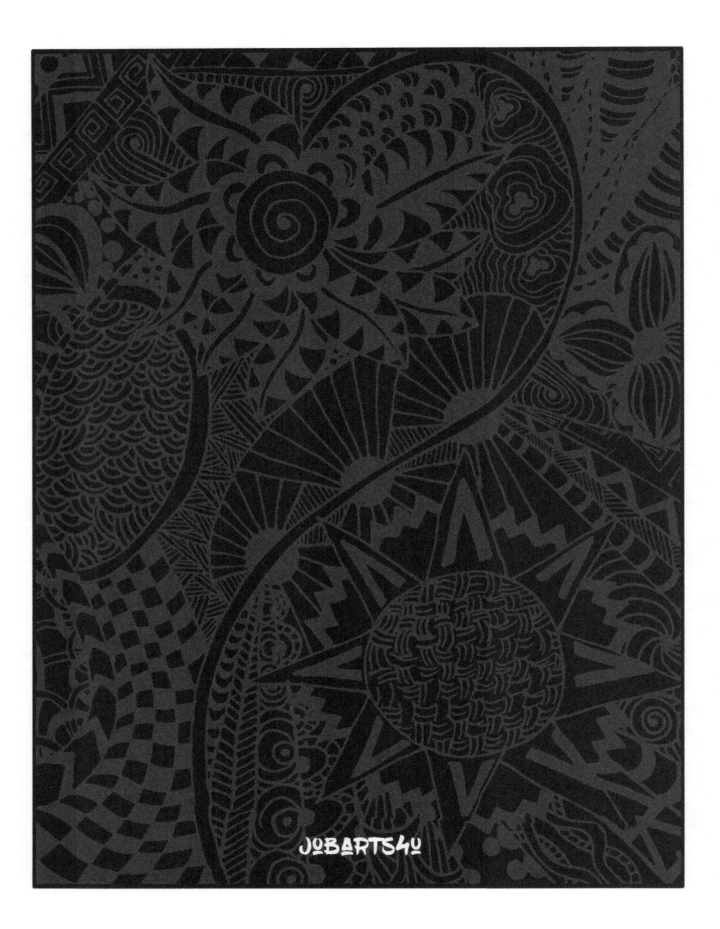

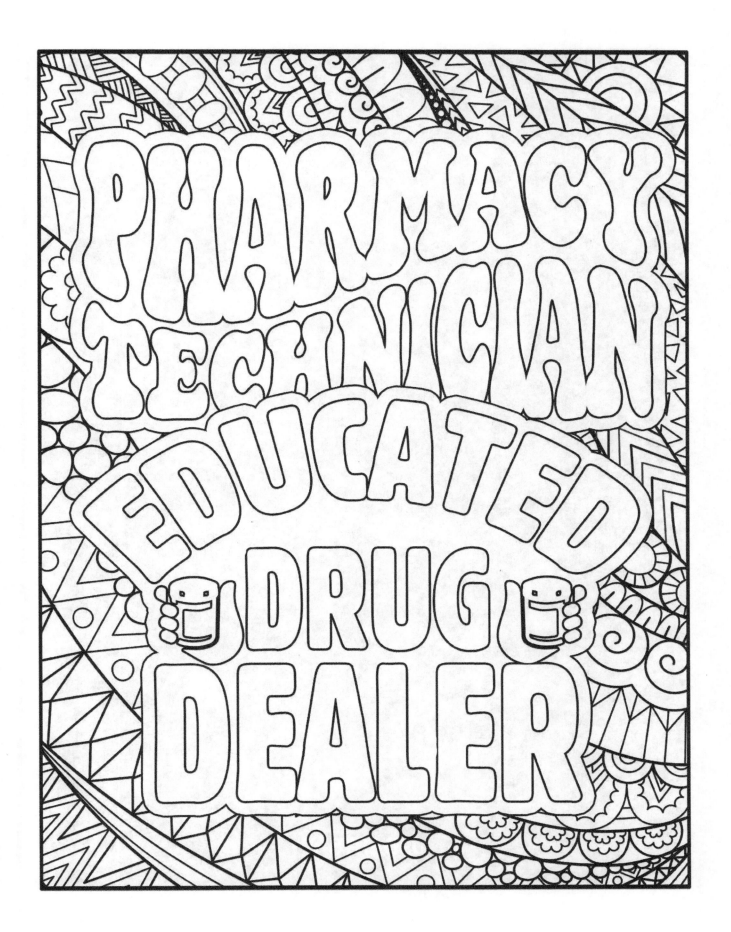

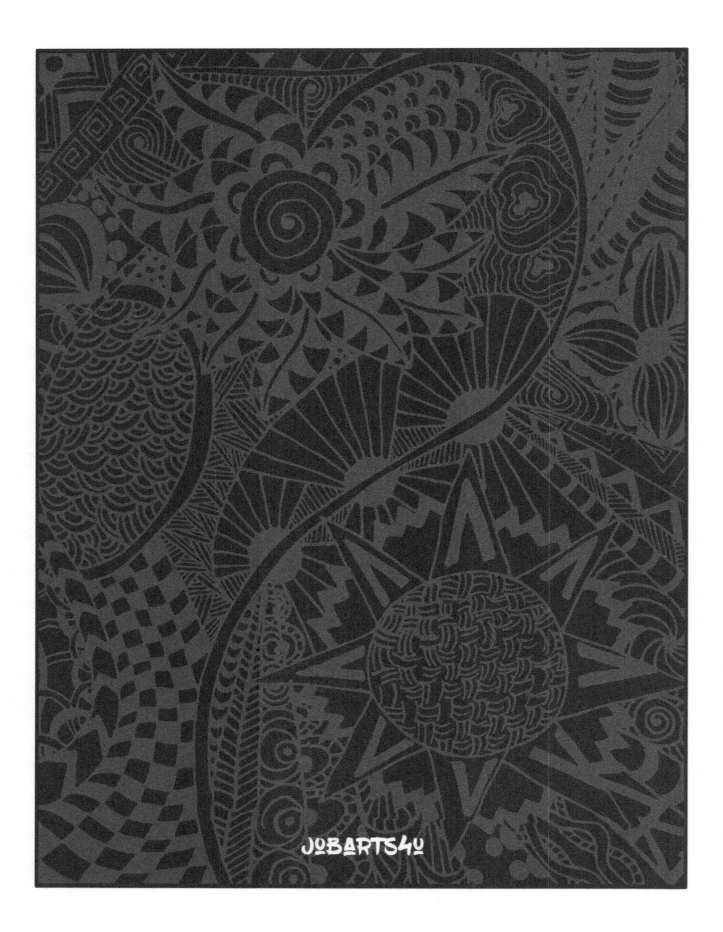

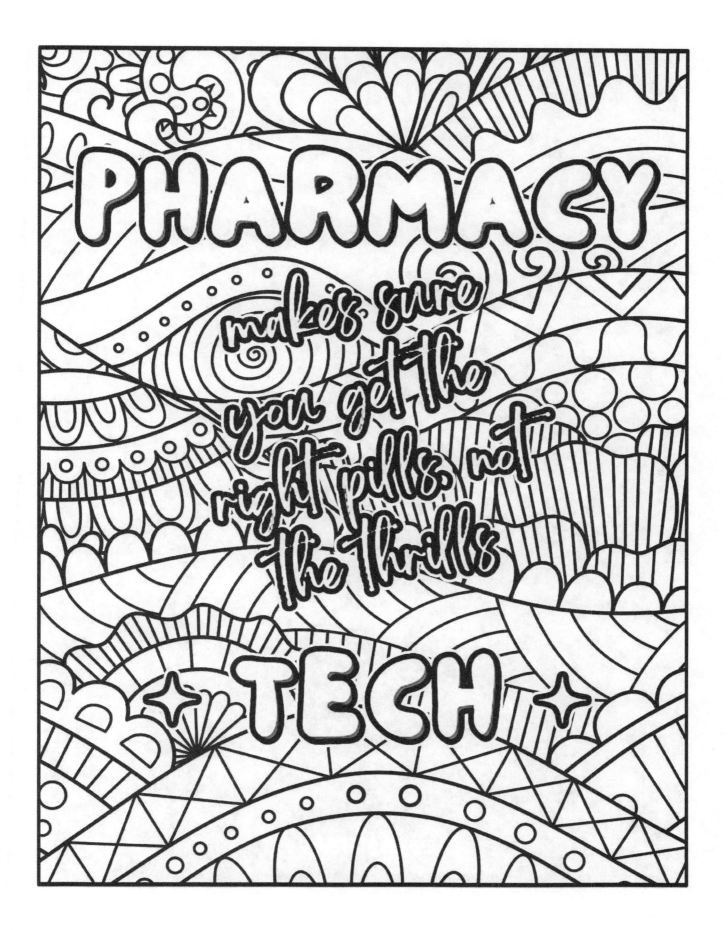

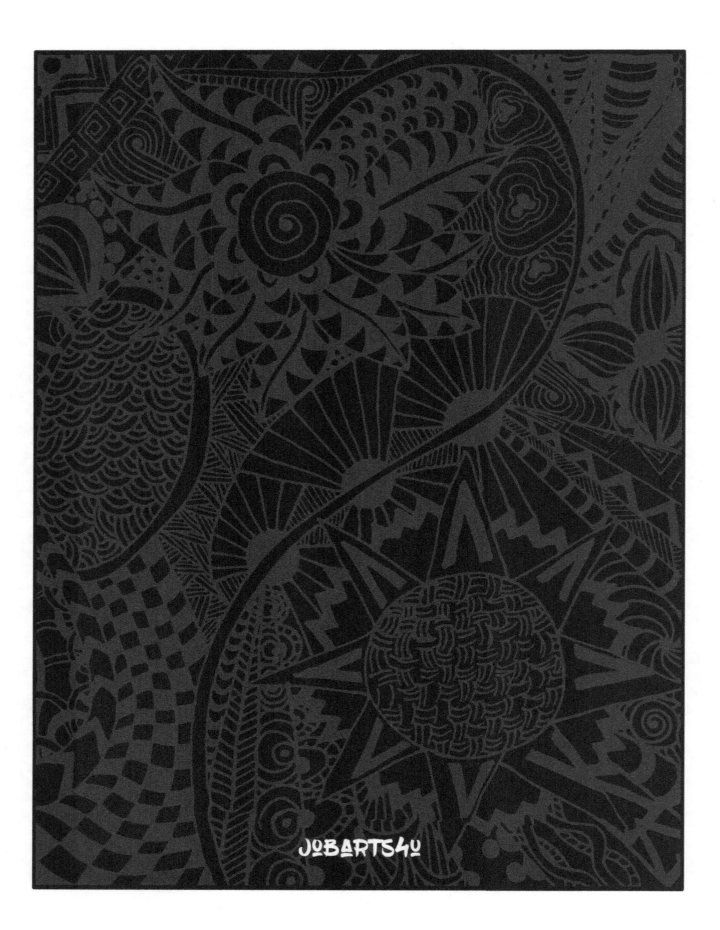

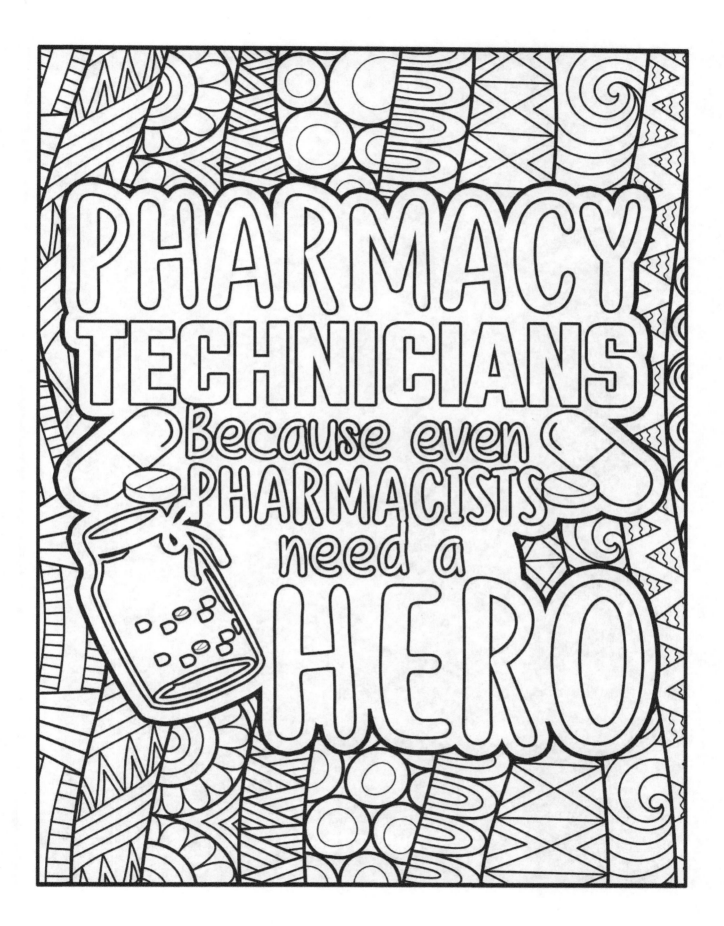

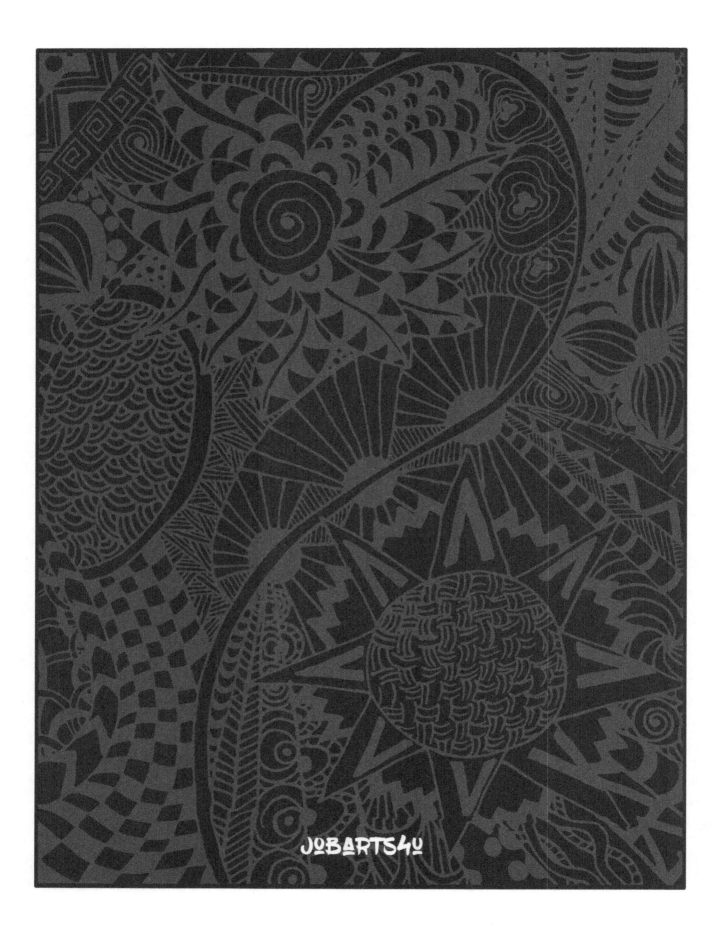

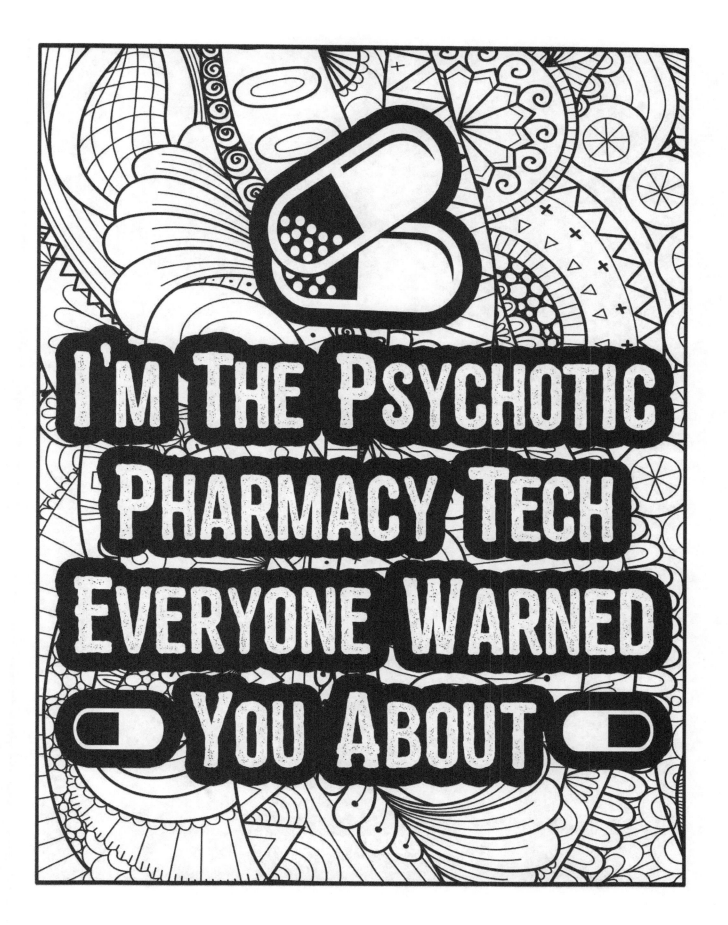

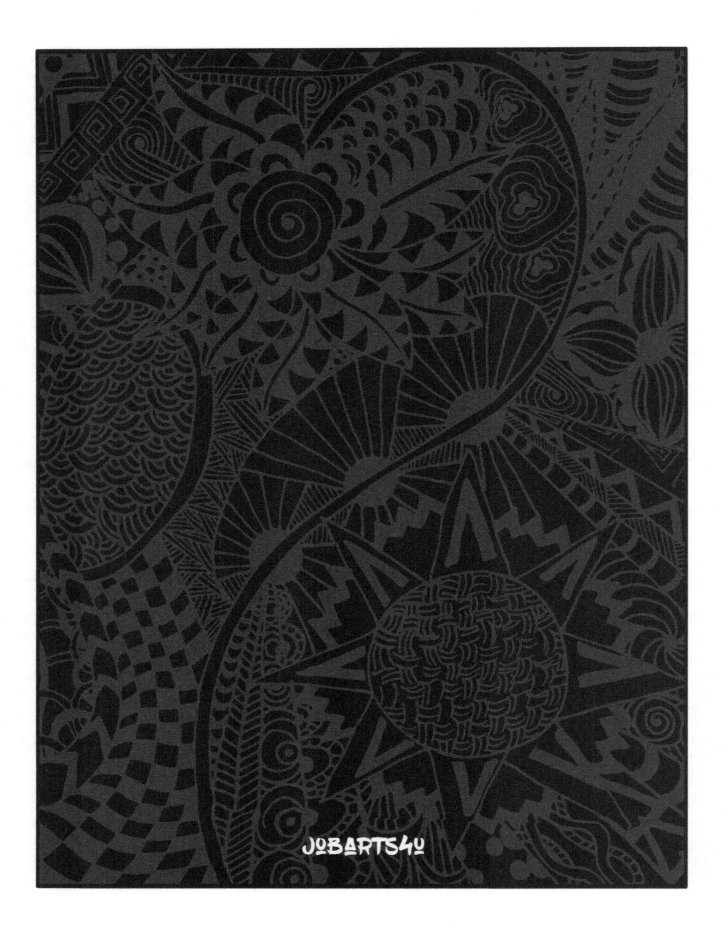

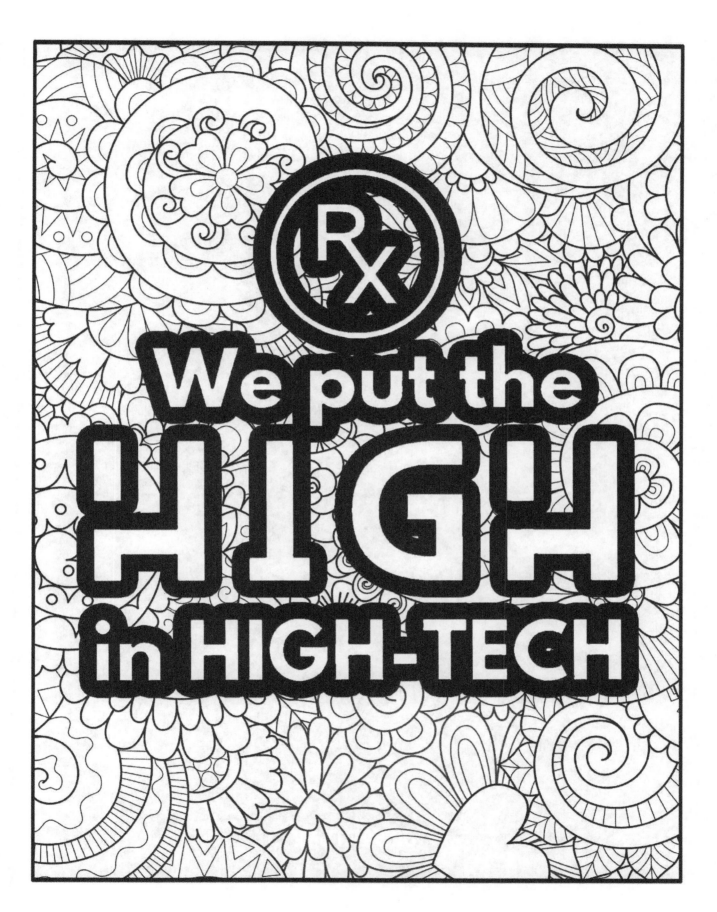

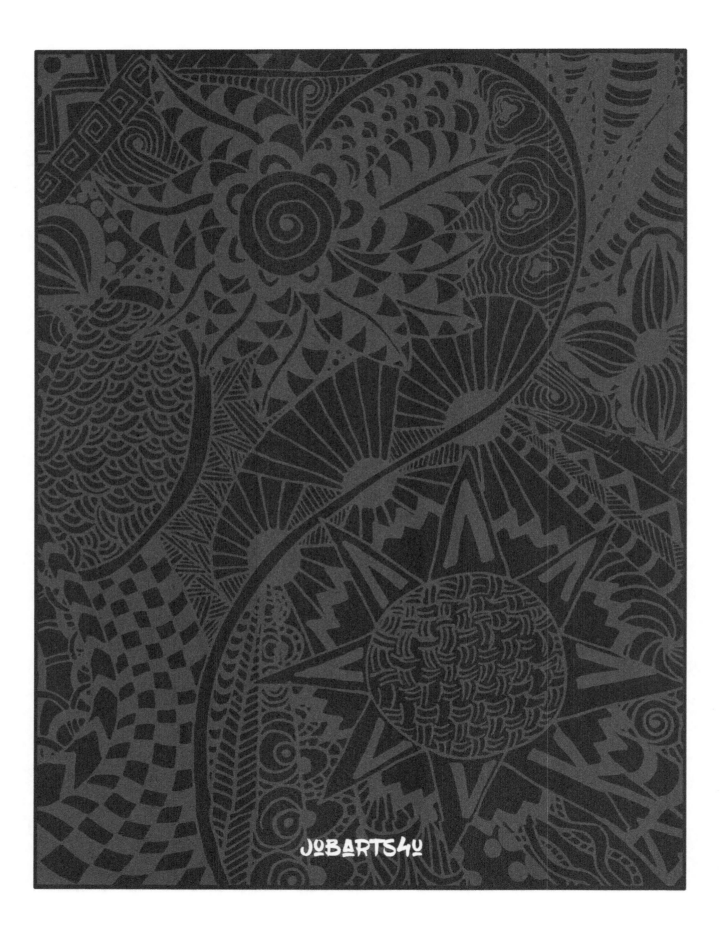

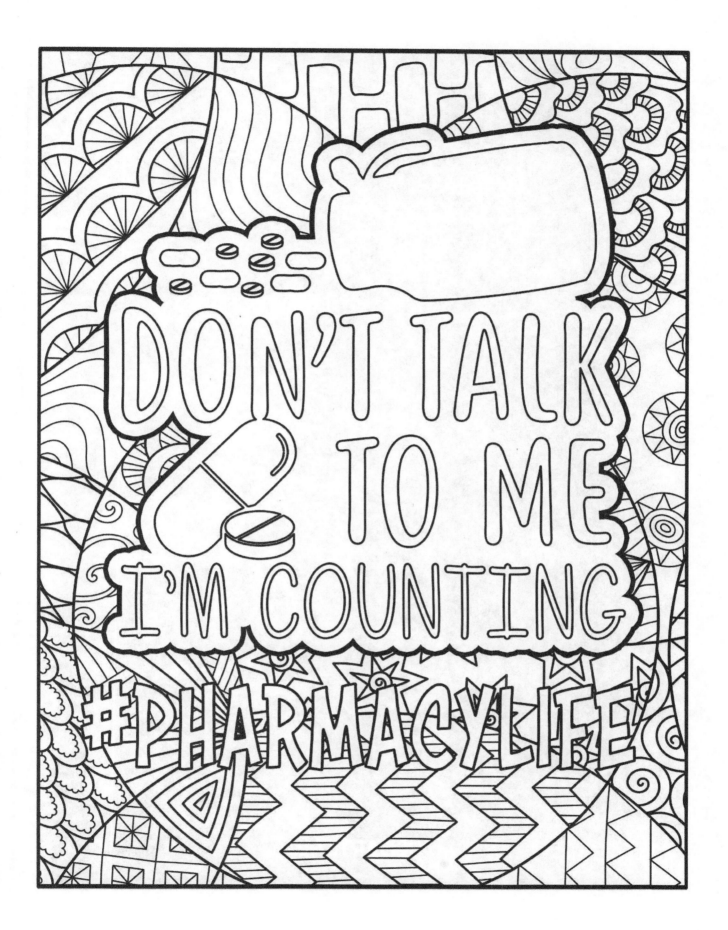

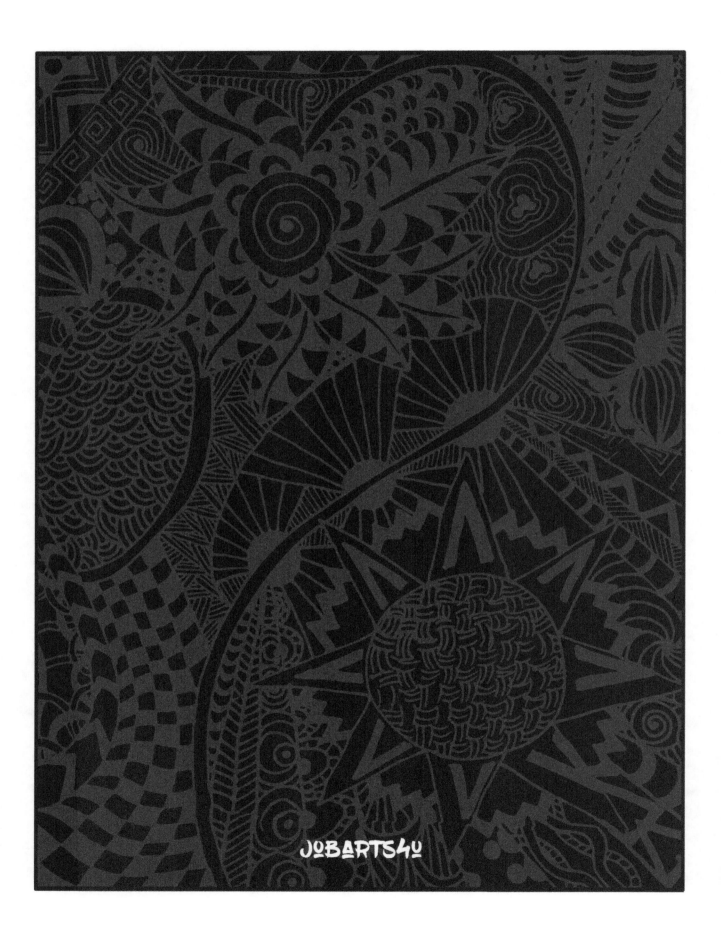

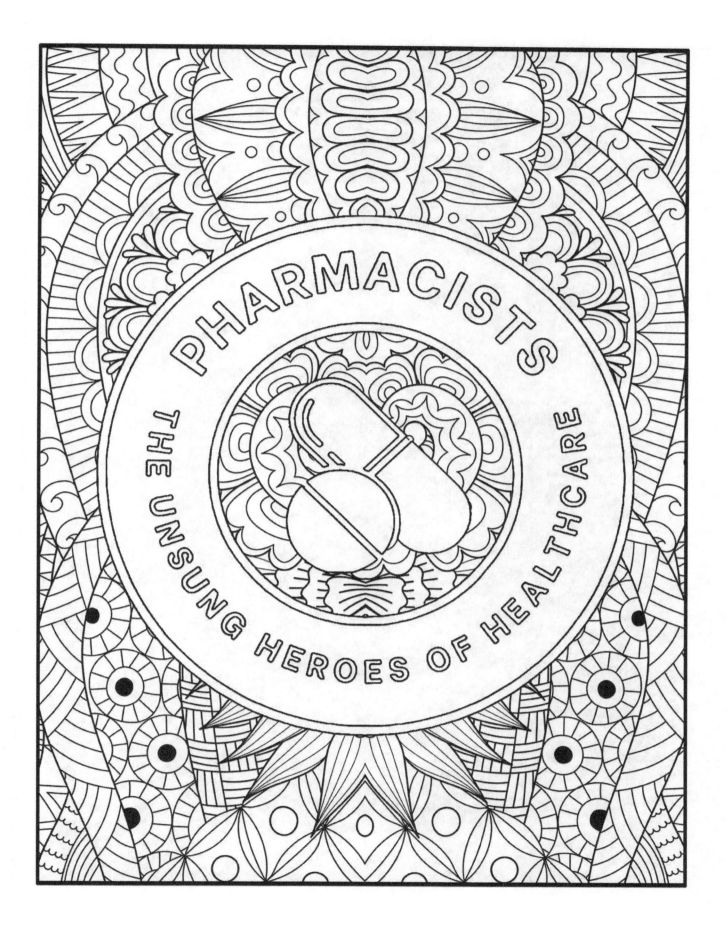

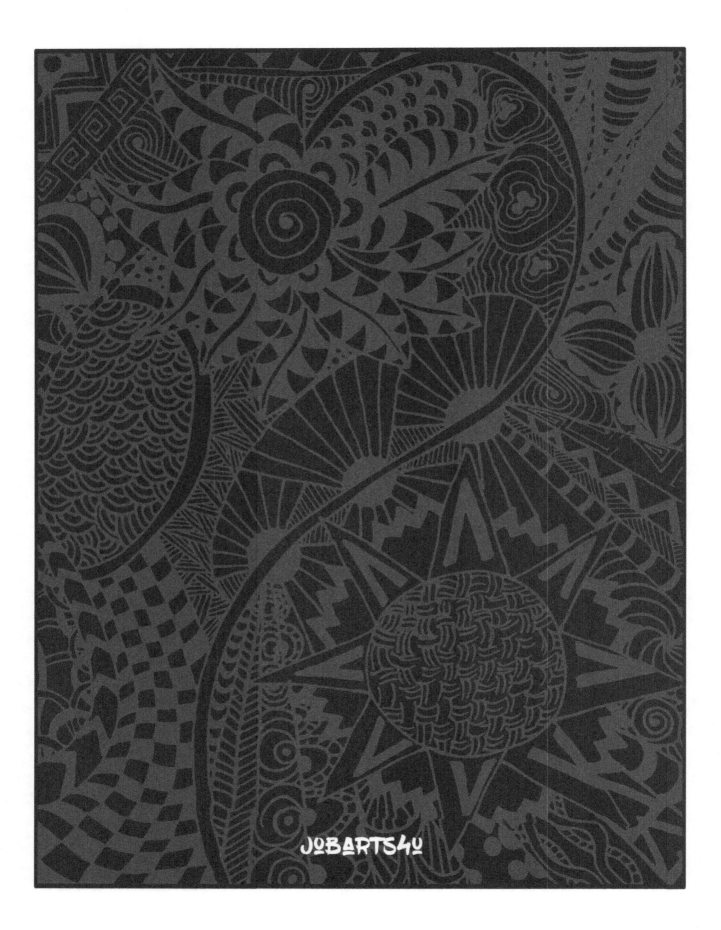

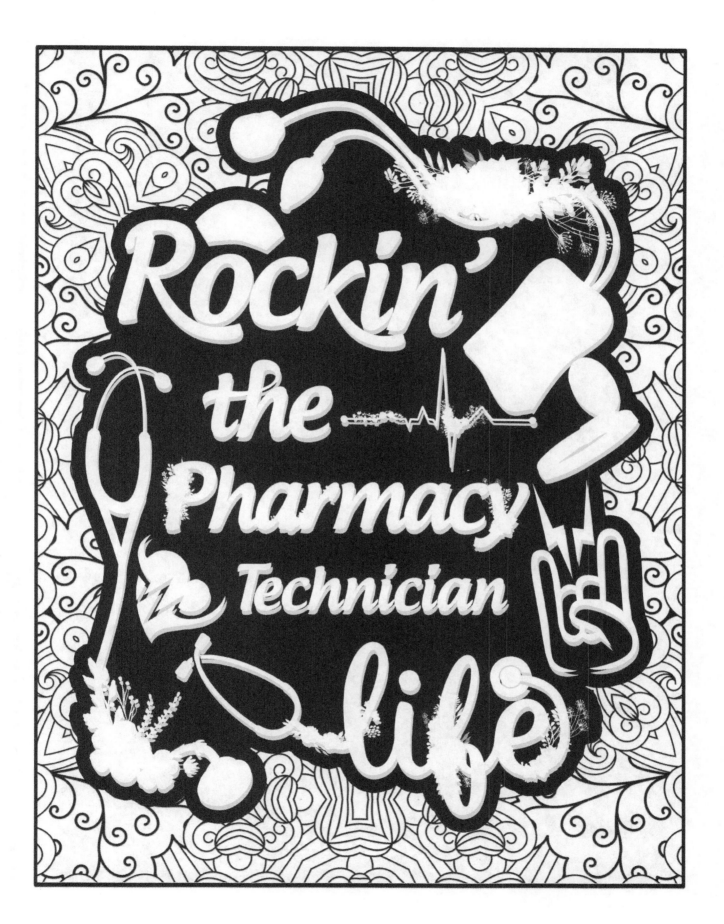

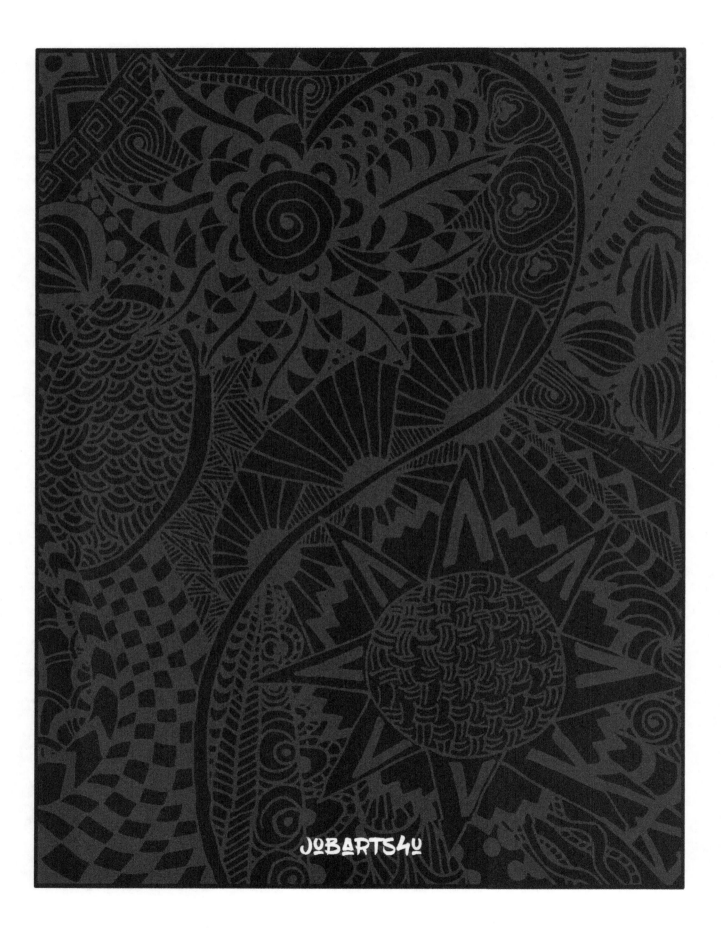

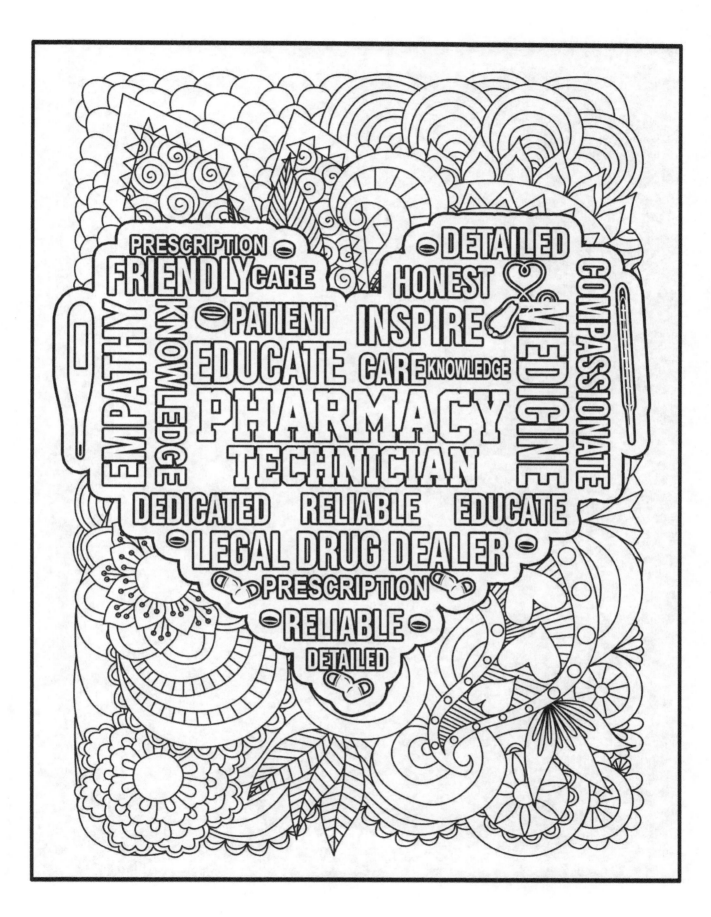

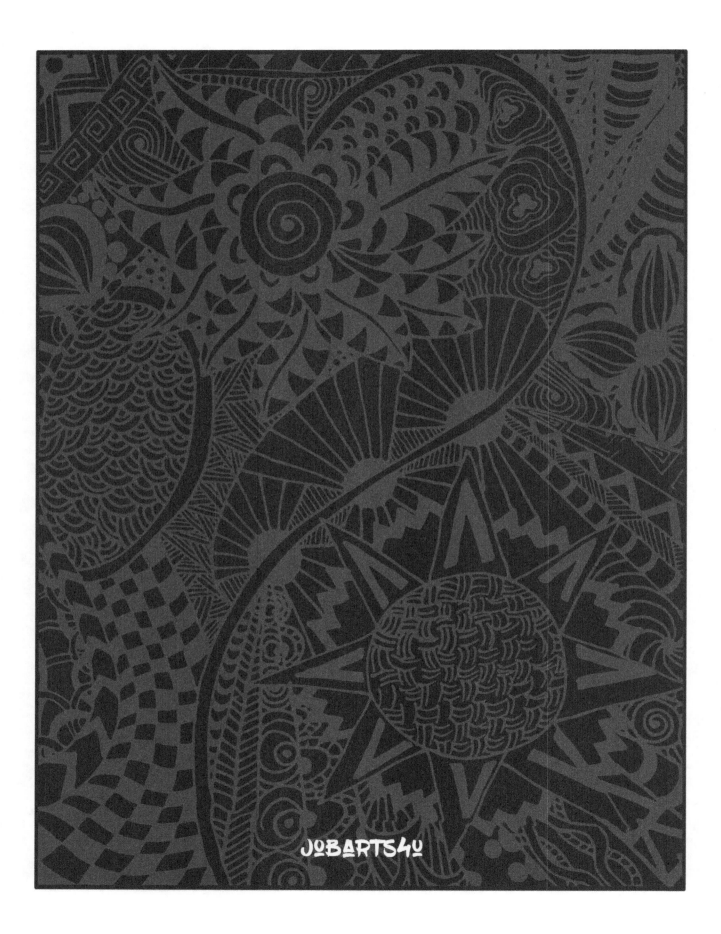

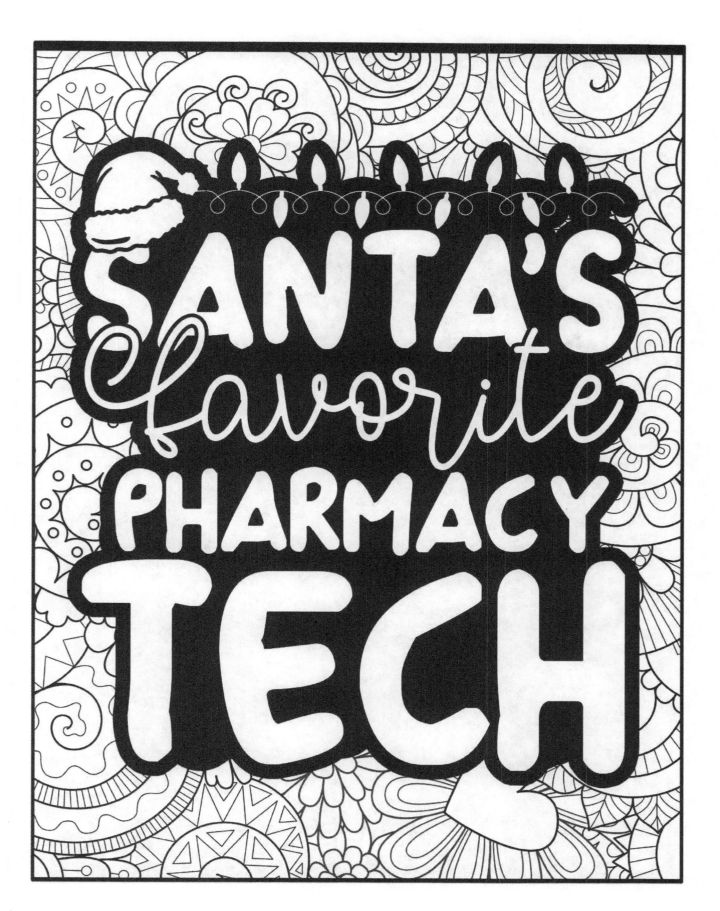

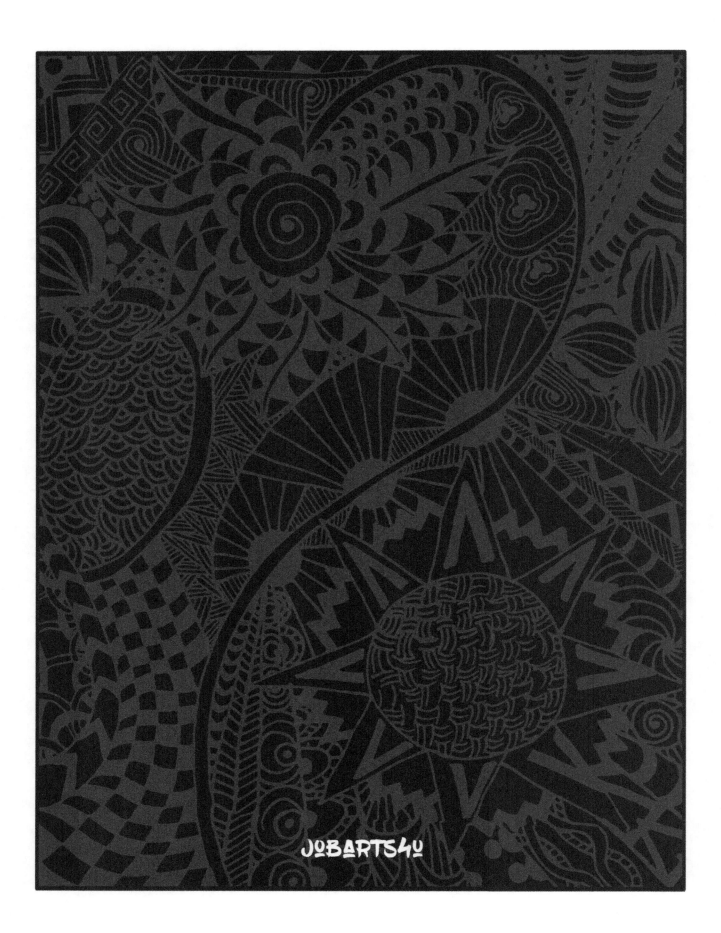

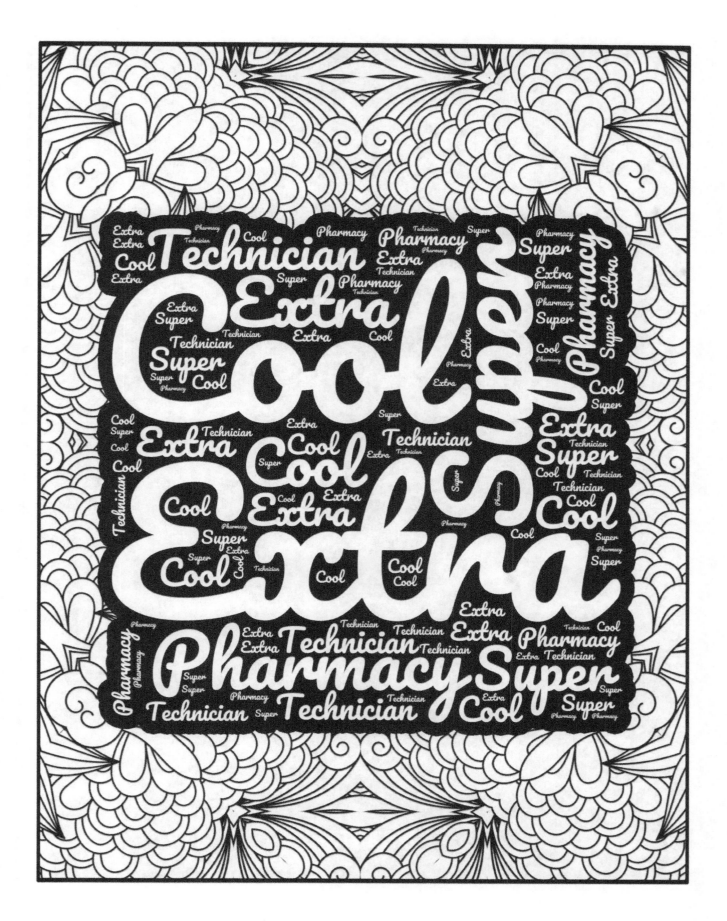

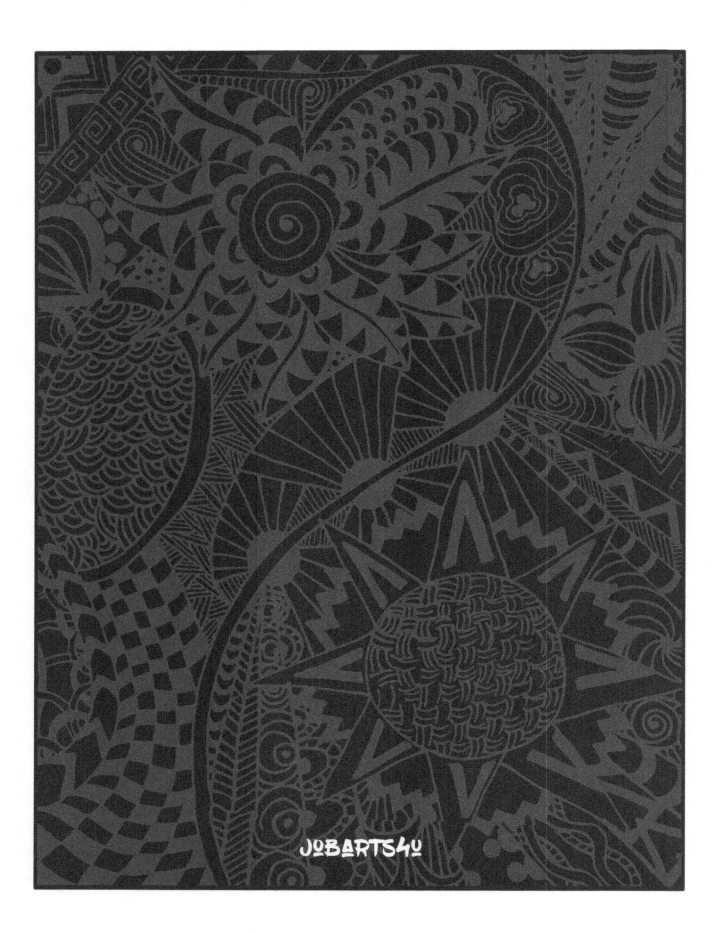

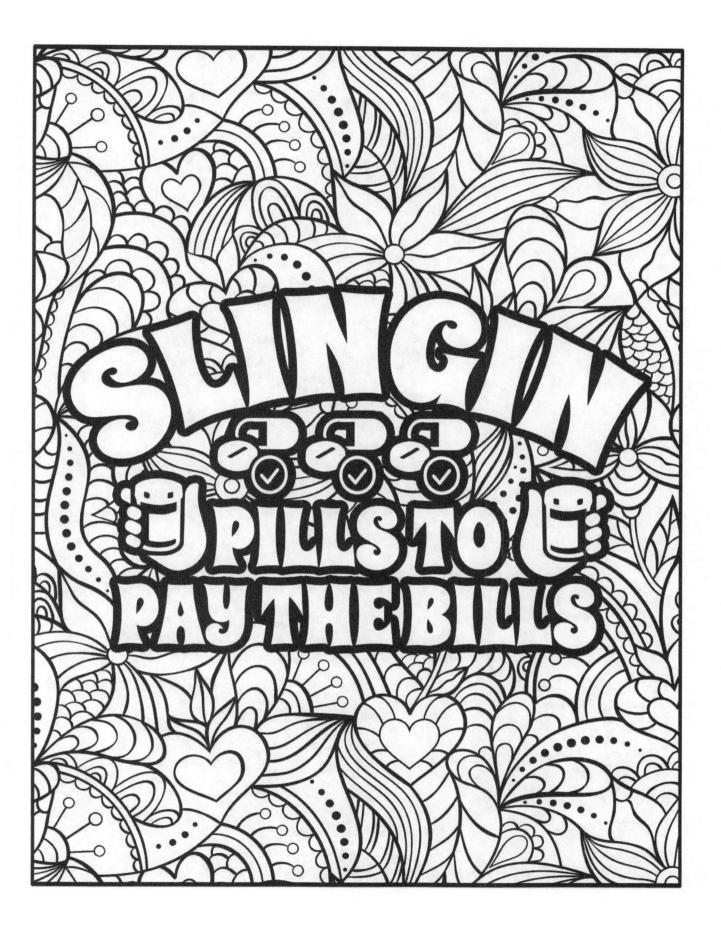

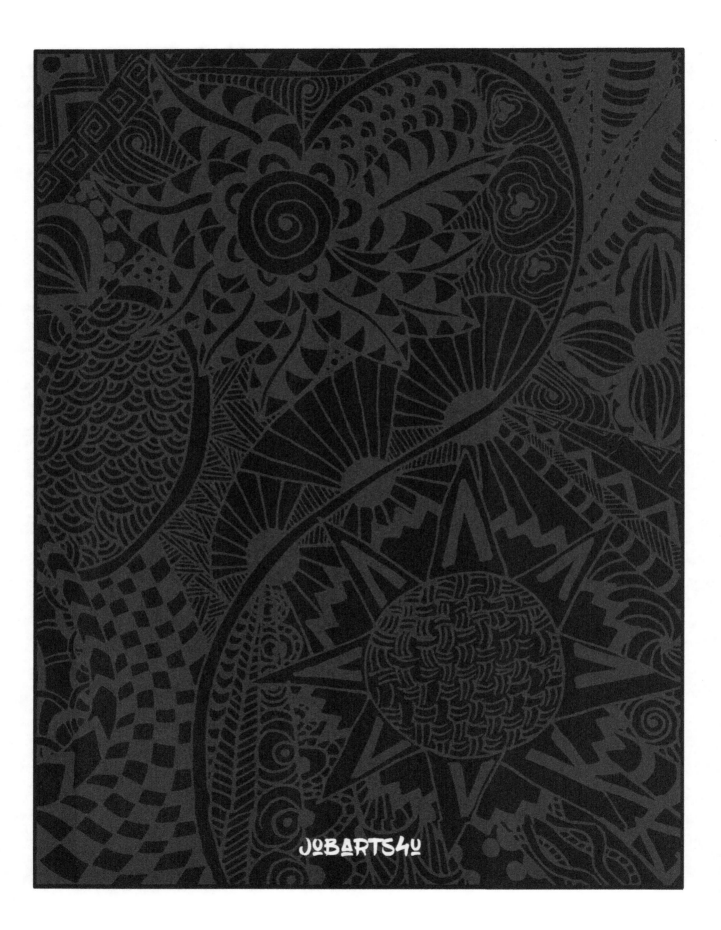

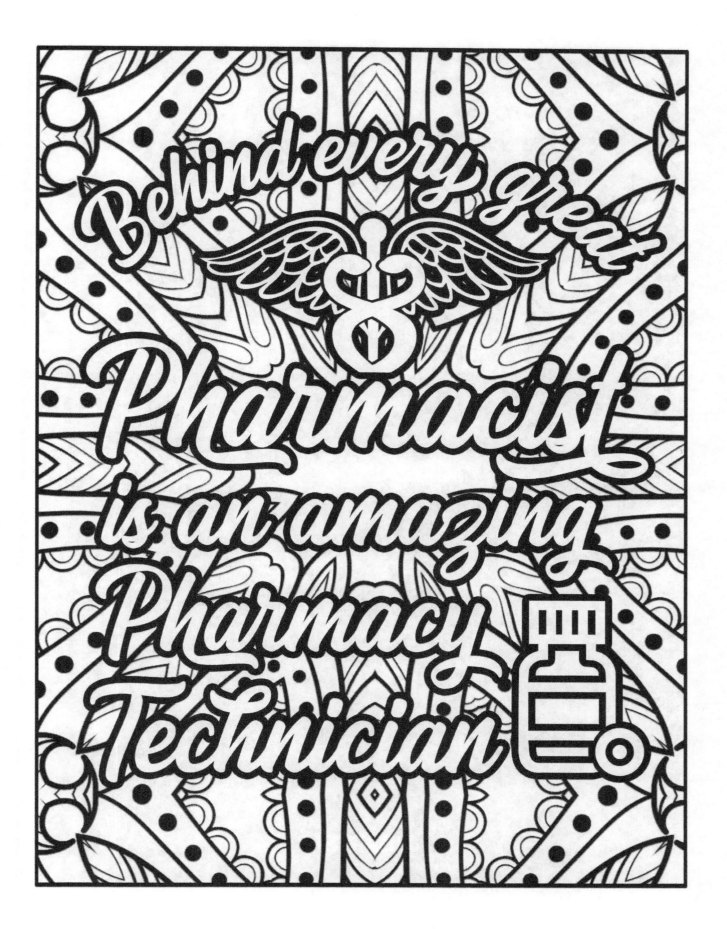

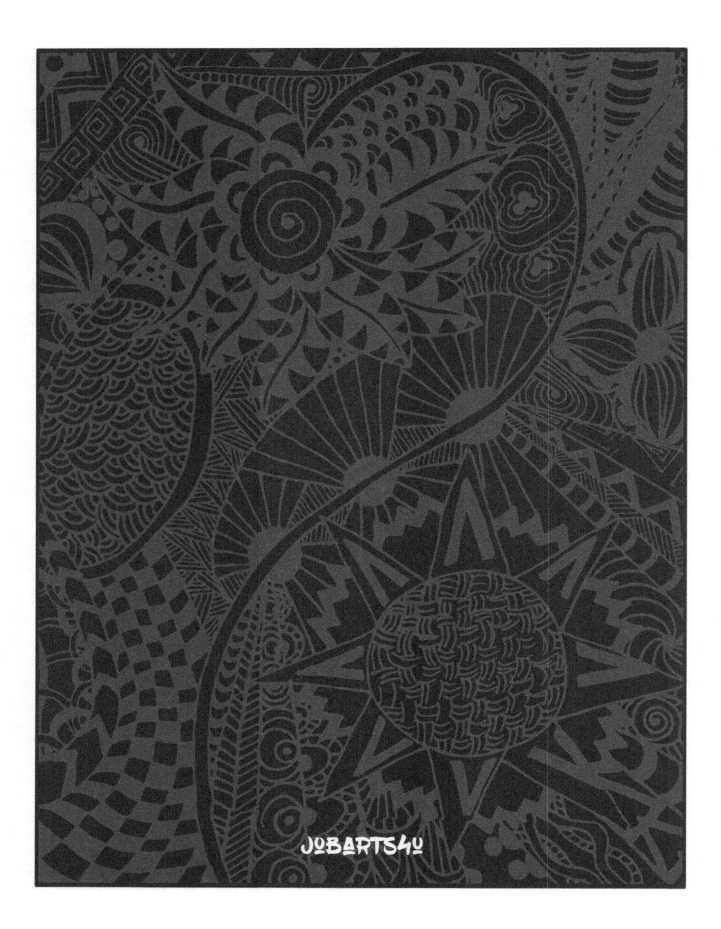

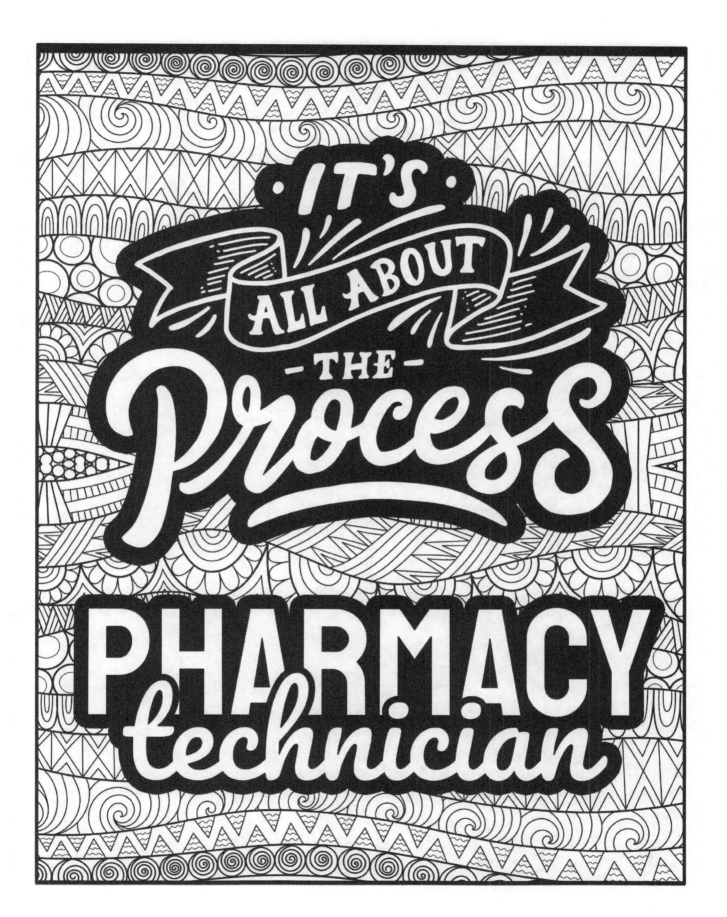

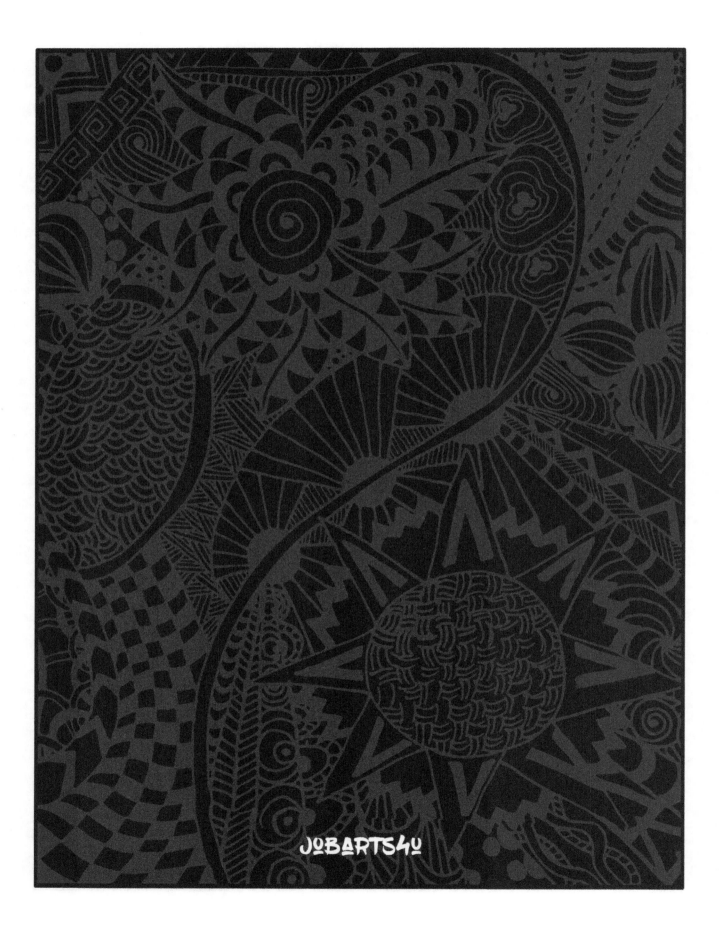

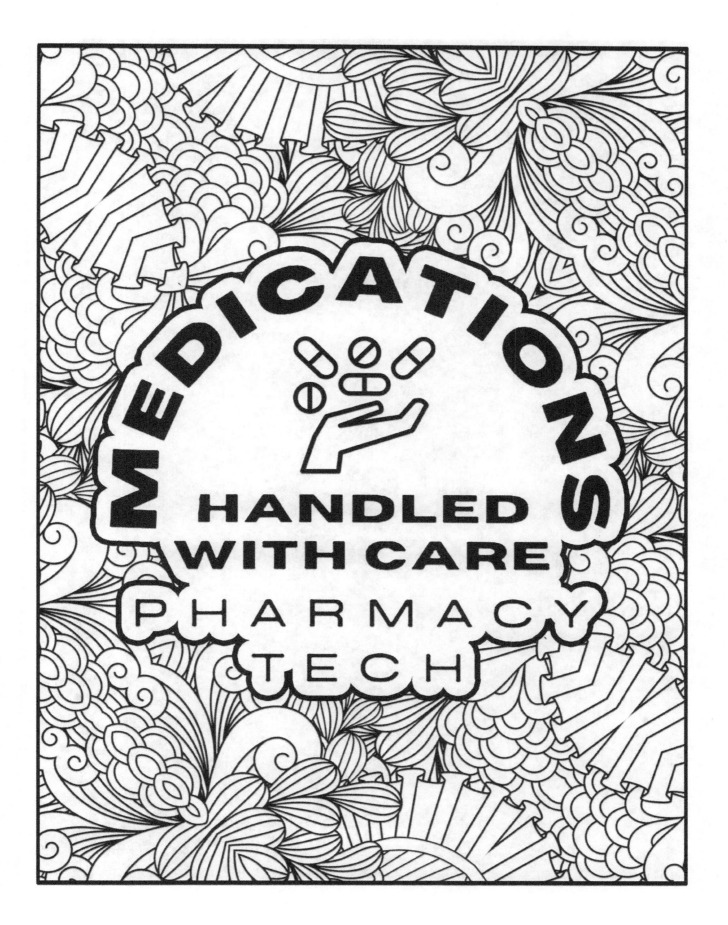

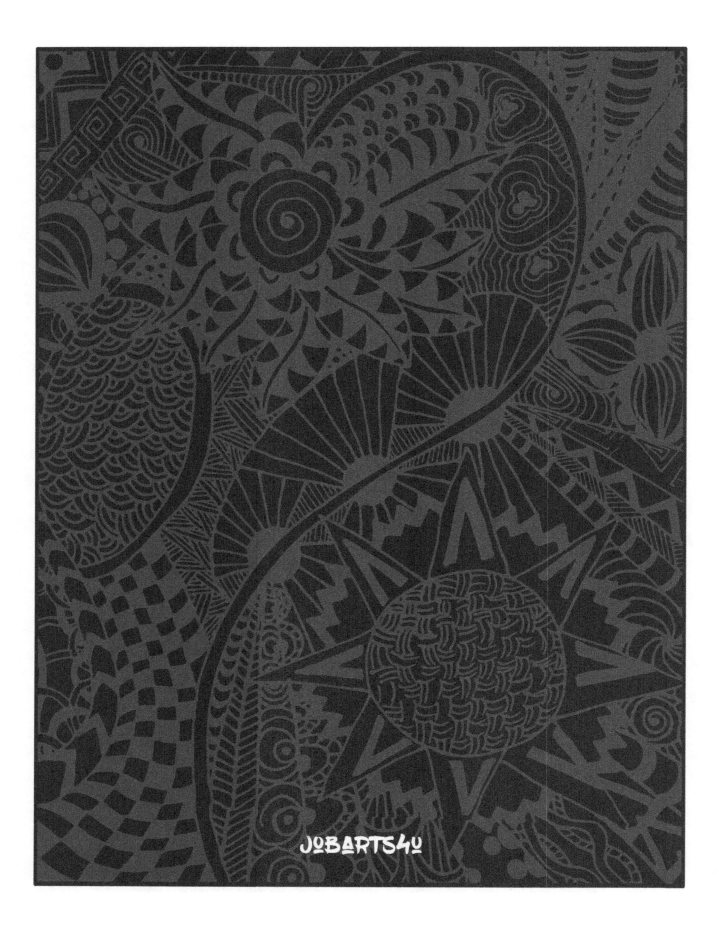

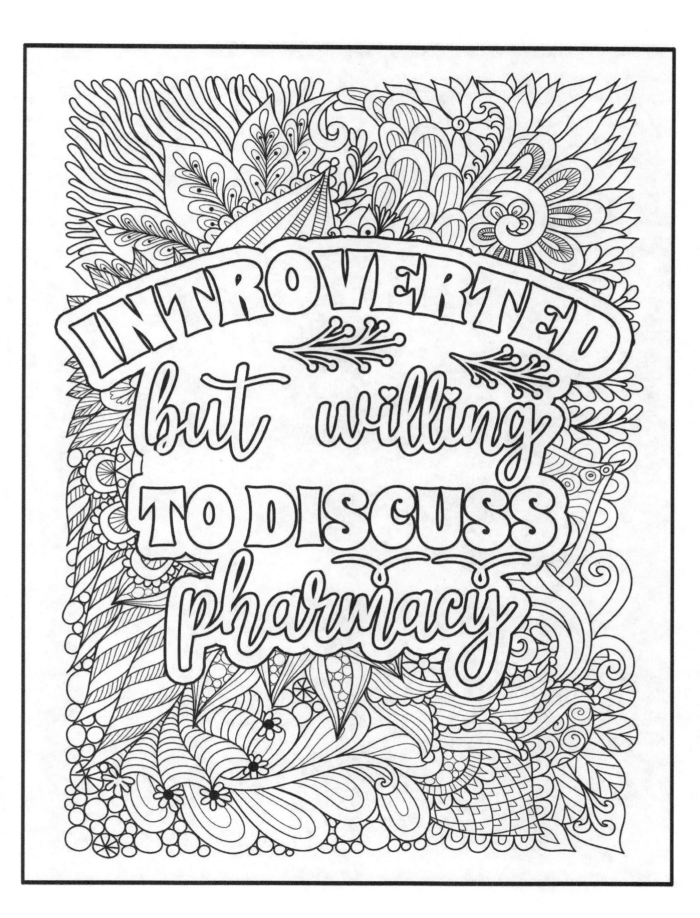

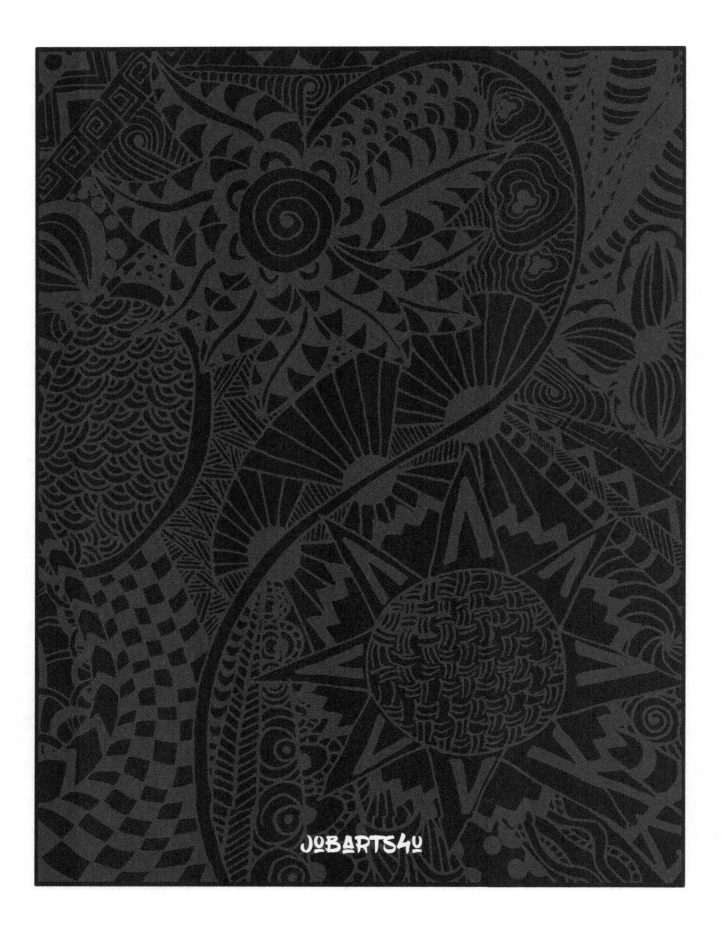

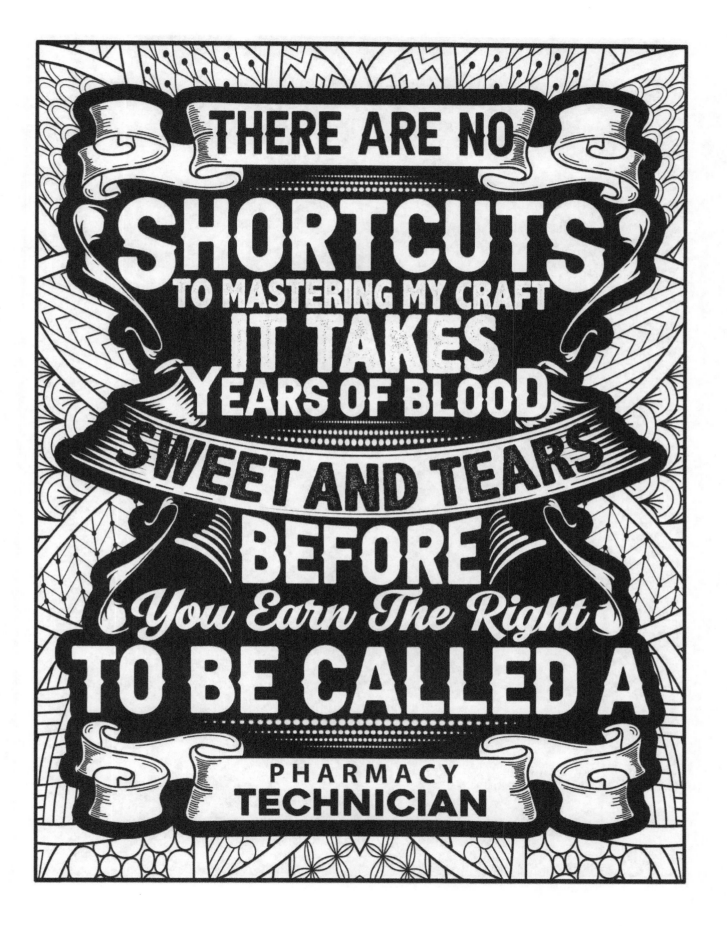

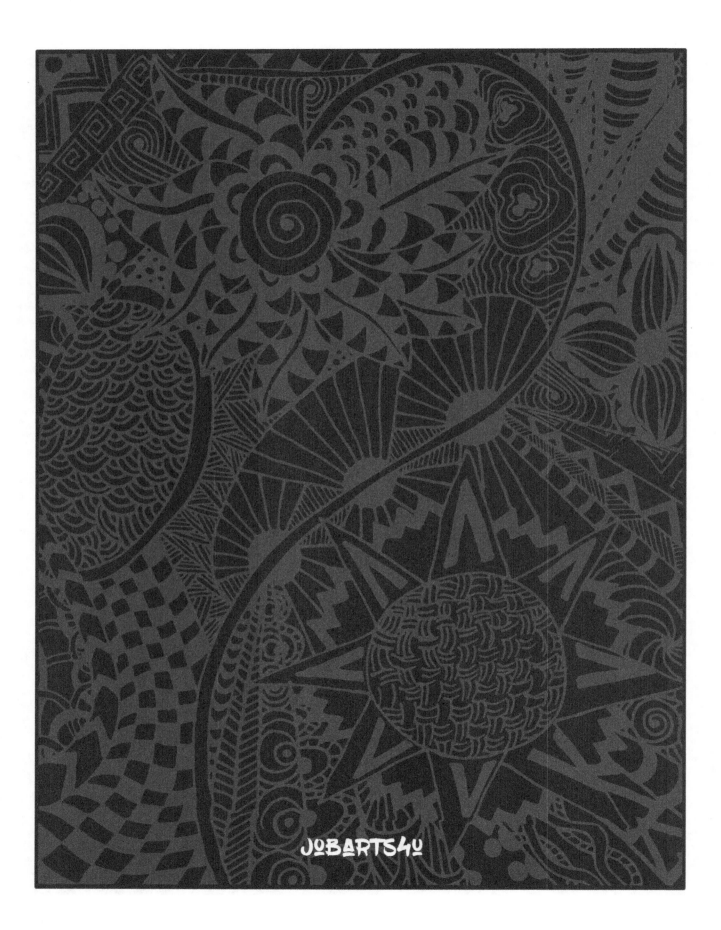

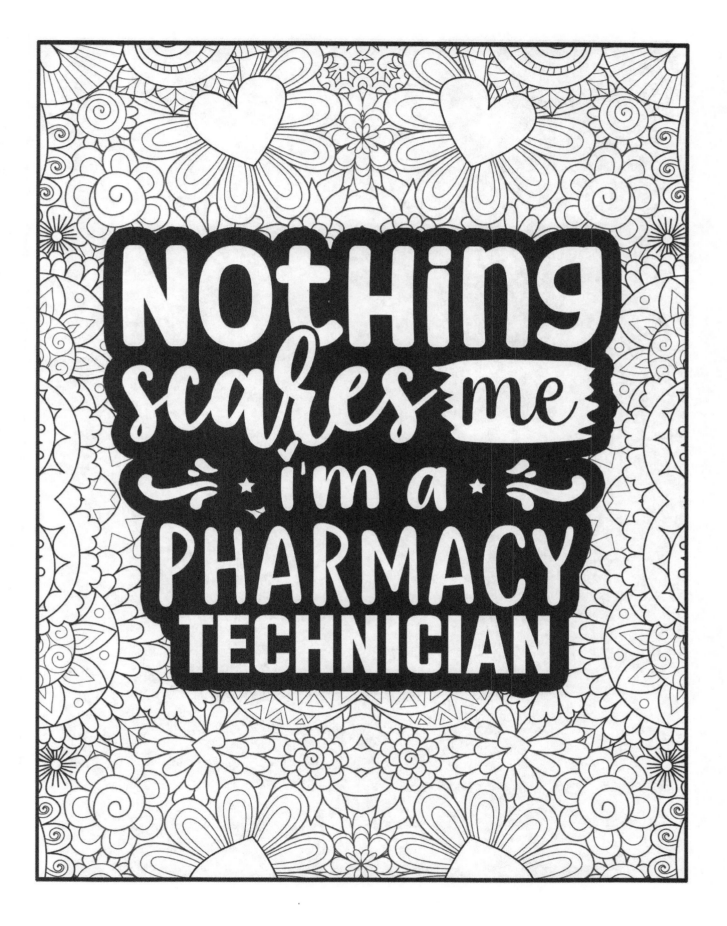

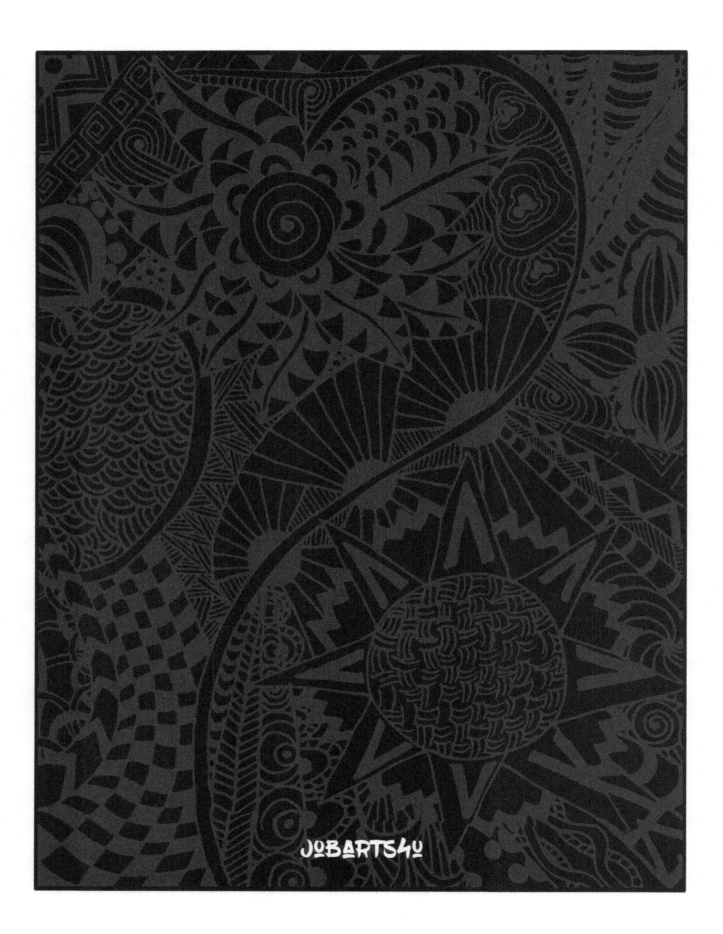

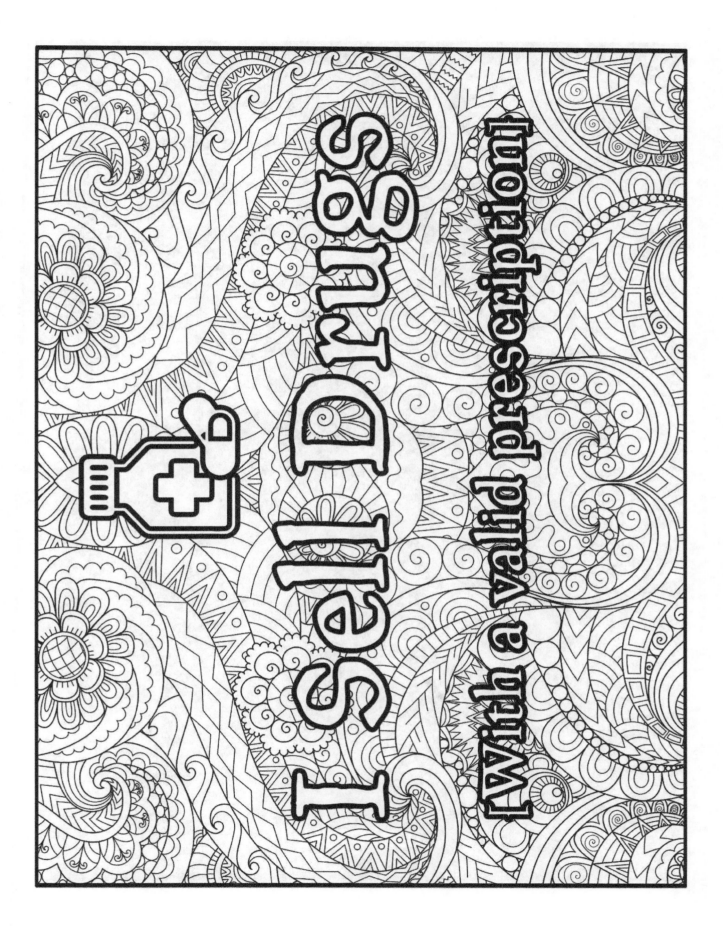

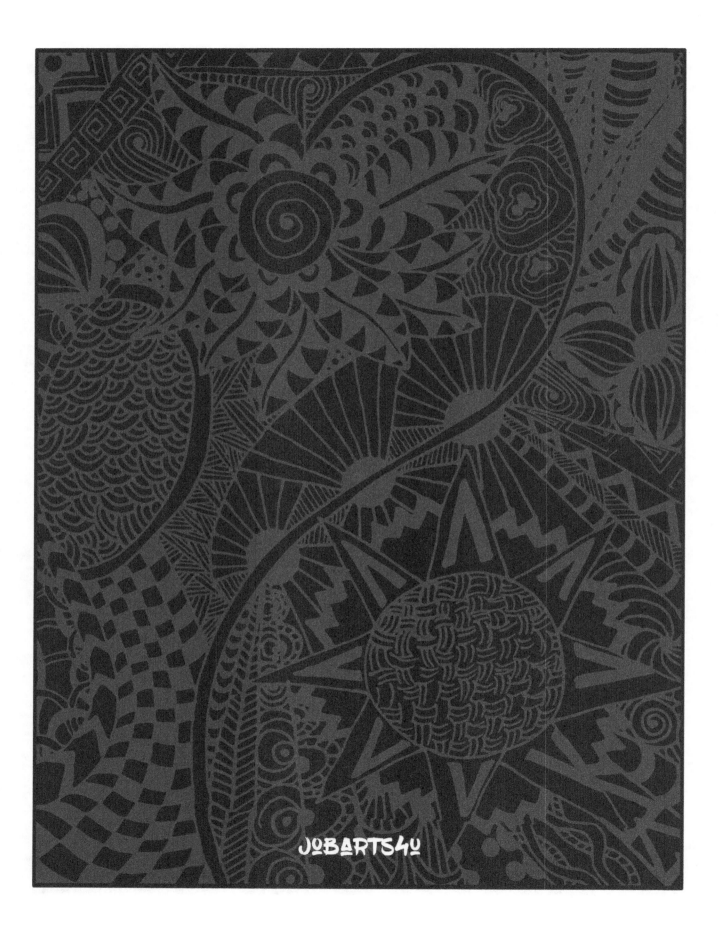

Made in United States
North Haven, CT
26 December 2024